WOMAN TO MOTHER

WOMAN • TO • MOTHER

A Transformation

Vangie Bergum

Foreword by Michel Odent

BERGIN & GARVEY PUBLISHERS, INC.
MASSACHUSETTS

First published in 1989 by
Bergin & Garvey Publishers, Inc.
670 Amherst Road
Granby, Massachusetts 01033

90   987654321

Printed in the United States of America

Library of Congress Cataloging-in-Publication Data

Bergum, Vangie.
    Woman to mother; a transformation / Vangie Bergum.
        p. cm.
    Bibliography: p.
    Includes index.
    ISBN 0–89789–183–X (alk. paper): $34.95
    ISBN 0–89789–182–1 (pbk.: alk. paper): $12.95
    1. Motherhood.   2. Pregnancy—Psychological aspects.
    3. Childbirth—Psychological aspects.   4. Mother and child.
    I. Title.
    HQ759.B465 1988
    306.8'743—dc19   88-26061
                                                          CIP

"Elsa's Birth," pp. 138–39, is excerpted with permission from Jessica Murray and
Mothering Magazine, Mother Poet, published by John McMahon and Peggy
O'Mara McMahon, P.O. Box 1690, Santa Fe, N.M. 87504. All rights reserved.

Parts of Chapter 5 first appeared in Vangie Kelpin (Bergum), "Birthing Pain,"
Phenomenology + Pedagogy 2(2): 178–87. Used with permission of the editor.

For mothers

In memory of my mother, Edna Bergum Vinge

And daughters

For my daughter, Siri Nina Bergum Kelpin

Contents

Foreword

"So, Amanda, now you are a mother."
Amanda replied with a smile. In her smile I saw a complex mixture of joy, awareness, wisdom, self-respect, and a sense of responsibility.
This had been our only conversation during the hour following the birth of Amanda's baby girl. Amanda was still seated on the floor of her bathroom, holding the baby in her arms.

As soon as I was back home after this birth, I had a look at my mail. A manuscript. A title: *Woman to Mother. A Transformation*.

I have read many books about pregnancy, childbirth, being in the womb, being born, being a mother, being a father . . . but I have never read any study focusing on this magical transformation, this mutation I have witnessed thousands of times. This transformation which urges one to say: "Now, you are a mother."

There are two important times when you make your opinion about a book. The first one is when you read the title. The second is when you read the first sentence you come across by opening the book at random. Right away I came across this sentence, "Giving birth changes how you see the world."

What do we need urgently at the end of this century? What do we need in a male dominated society which is destroying the planet at an uncontrolled speed?

We need to change how we see the world. We need to develop our capacity to see far away in the future. We need to see the planet as a living creature we are responsible for. We need to learn responsibility.

This is exactly what a woman learns as soon as she becomes a mother. This is what humanity as a whole has to learn.

The book by Vangie Bergum comes at a time when we need a feminine attitude towards the planet earth. It comes at a time when we need the reintegration of specifically feminine values.

This book is a necessary contribution to "the return of the Goddess."

—Michel Odent

Preface

"Becoming a mother is an inner journey for women," says author Vangie Bergum. "Of course, it is an outer one too—marked by the burgeoning waist, the ballooning clothes, the awkward gait, and for many, a radiant and wholesome face." In this book Vangie Bergum sets out to describe "the integrated reality" of both this outer and inner process. She aims to make available to us the lived meanings of the transformative moments that women experience as they become mothers through desiring, bearing, birthing, and caring for children.

In many ways this is a book about beginnings. It is about birth, the beginning of new life for every person. It is also about becoming a mother, the birth of a new life for a woman. This book itself is a beginning. It is the beginning of a quest for the meaning of that unexplained chasm between the life of woman and the life of mother. There are books on women and there are books on mothering but few, if any, have been written, like this one, on the transformation of one into the other. Importantly, this book is the birth also of an author—the beginning of a wonderfully sensitive, simple, and strong voice.

I say "simple" not, of course, because this text is simplistic or naive. On the contrary this book somehow is able to treat something complex and deep—the transformation of woman to mother—in an intelligible and whole manner. The word "simple" originally means "undivided, together, whole." An approach that is "simple" aims to ward off the pulverizing pressures of using an interest in life as a pretext for escaping from the wholeness of the lived world—fragmenting abstractions of theories about life. Those involved in the social and human sciences know that it is often more demanding to say something worth saying while staying close to life than it is to theorize and formulate abstractions about life.

And with this point we have arrived at another sense in which this book is concerned with beginnings. As we read the life stories of Brenda, Christine, Jane, Susan, Anna, and Katherine, we become aware that with each story— and with each subsequent interpretation of their transformative meanings— Vangie Bergum is exploring the living contours of beginnings. Each chapter is thus a study of beginnings: in the section on "the decision" to have a child she searches for the beginnings of the transformative process; in "the body with child" she finds in the blood mystery the dawn of the maternal relation; in "the pain of birthing" she shows how the experience of pain makes a new beginning possible—as the woman gives birth to the child, so the child in a sense births the mother; and in the chapters on the emerging "sense of responsibility" and "the experience of living with a child on one's mind" Vangie Bergum searches for the nascent sense of the Other as a prologue to a renewed sense of self—the woman as mother of the child; and so forth.

By constantly going back to beginnings, Vangie Bergum develops her own method of inquiry. This is not the methodological structure of a logocentric argument, aiming to nail down the meaning of birthing within a narrow feminist or theoretical medical discourse. Rather, Vangie Bergum's method is cyclical, more essentially feminist at heart. She attempts ever and anew to rid herself of conceptual wrappings and theoretical assumptions by beginning again and again with the narrative of lived life itself. *Woman to Mother: A Transformation* is also, or maybe especially, a book that explores what it means to be a woman in a modern society that has witnessed liberating forces, as well as destructive assaults on traditional rationalities, gender roles, and institutions such as the family. "Feminine" originally meant Mother: "she who suckles." Therefore, to search the beginnings of the meanings of mother is simultaneously a search for the fundamental meanings of femininity.

There are many voices in this book. At one level there are the representatives of the medical profession, academics, nurses, midwives, feminists, fathers, children, and foremost, the voices of the six women/mothers around whom this interpretive study evolves. At a second level there is the voice of the author. Vangie Bergum engages those various voices by attentively listening to them and by being sensitive to what these voices allow women to hear and how they allow women to come to certain self-understandings of the transformative experience of birth in a broad sense. At no point is the voice of the author intrusive or polemical toward the conversational partners she engages. This I believe is indicative of the strength of Vangie Bergum's commitment to a feminist principle: to foster a thoughtfulness that is integrative, imaginative, relational, intuitive, and visionary—oriented toward experiences that are sentient, whole, unifying, vital, and cyclical in their value to life. There are few, if any, hard lines in this book. In thinking about the implications of her text for health professionals Vangie Bergum weighs the metaphors of the deconstructive power of Nietzsche's hammer against the healing potential of Florence Nightingale's lamp. She allows for the need of health professionals to battle the oppressive symbolic and institutional structures of traditional medicine in order for the light of true healing to be possible.

Throughout this book Vangie Bergum brings the reader into a conversational relationship with the question: What is the nature of the transformation of woman to mother? The partners she chooses for this conversational relation, and the situations and events she wants us to discuss, are cause of sure controversy. But it is by virtue of her own strong voice that the conversation she leads, with her partners and with us her readers, never closes down into a self-serving polemic. There is much that women and mothers, health professionals and educators, men and fathers can learn from the conversational form and content of this wonderful text.

—Max van Manen

Acknowledgments

This work would never have been undertaken or accomplished without the support of family, friends, colleagues, and, most importantly, the women who talked with me during the period of this study. Although the research was initiated and completed as a requirement for a graduate study program, the impact for me has been much broader than the scholarly endeavor.

Being a woman and a mother gave me the actuality from which to begin to think about the experience of becoming a mother as a transforming one. My experience being mother to my son, Sem, and my daughter, Siri, is the reality from which the desire to explore this phenomenon originated. I want to acknowledge, with thankfulness, these teenage children as being at the very heart of this work. Brault Kelpin, my husband and parenting partner, supported me in this labor as he did in my birthing labors. His caring words and actions assisted in clarifying my thinking, calming my turmoiled spirit, guiding my use of technology, and steadfastly reminding me of my task. I could not have accomplished this project without his involvement. I want to thank my family for their care and understanding, especially Dorothy Engen, Nina and Percy Bergquist, and Paul and Merry Kelpin.

My research advisor, Max van Manen, listened, prodded, challenged, disagreed, supported, and enhanced the ideas explored throughout this study. This book reflects my association with him—his interest in this work and his persistent encouragement have affected me deeply.

Ted Aoki, Robert Burch, Amy Zelmer, Dyanne Affonso, Peggy-Anne Field, Terrance Carson, Carol Olson, Angeline Martel, Rod Evans, Jane Ross, and Madeleine Grumet are thanked for reading and commenting on various parts of this work. To have Michel Odent comment in the Foreword is an honor. Special thanks to Jean Ure, and to Ottilie Sanderson, Carla Novikoff, Laura Hargrave, and Ann Lever who assisted me in concrete ways.

Of course, the women who shared their experiences of becoming mothers are the main contributors to this work. Brenda, Christine, Anna, Jane, Susan, and Katherine gave generously of their time, thoughts, and feelings, for which I have great respect and appreciation. The experiences of many other women (particularly Paula) also permeate the text: the willingness to share intimate vistas of individual lives is valued. Although the stories are based on particular women's "personal" lives, the comments and interpretations strive for an understanding that reflects "public" experiences shared by many women. I wish to thank all the women I have spoken with, read about, and observed during this study which gives me the opportunity to offer this view of women as mothers.

Acknowledgment is given to the Dr. Jean Nelson Memorial Foundation; the Alberta Foundation of Nursing Research; the Department of Secondary Education, University of Alberta; and the Alberta Association of Registered Nurses for financial support during parts of this research. The Faculty of Nursing, University of Alberta has also provided administrative assistance. These agencies and institutions are not necessarily supportive of the ideas or conclusions associated with this research. Rather, the ideas and meanings presented here reflect my understanding of women's experiences of becoming mothers. I am pleased that Jim Bergin of Bergin & Garvey Publishers expressed interest in publishing this work. My communications with him and Ann Gross, book editor, have been very cordial.

•

Chapter 1

In the Company of Women

W omen, today, live in a world of significant change, a world where their voices are penetrating a perpetual barrier of silence about women's experience. This is not because women are just now beginning to speak or because they now have something to say; they always have. It is not because now women's words are coming with clarity; for years women have spoken with profound depth and clear rationality about the world in which they live. It is not because they speak from a consensus of all women; women see the world from individual perspectives. Rather, it is that only now women are beginning to be heard. Perhaps there is increasing public recognition that our society will benefit from women's insight and knowledge (Morgan 1977, 1984). For whatever reason that women today speak, many are speaking about their social situations in the private realm (O'Brien 1981) and from a reality of childbearing and mothering (Chesler 1979). Whether or not the women who speak are actually mothers, the concerns are often centered around the "mother" aspect of women's lives (Daly 1978, 1984; Chicago

1985; O'Brien 1981). They speak to make their private worlds a public concern in areas such as equal pay for work of equal value, child care facilities, peace and nonviolence, human hospitals and home births, pro-choice or anti-abortion, pensions and family allowances, erotica rather than pornography, or sometimes simply for a woman to have "a room of [her] own."

There is a questioning by women of the relevance of male views of the world for women (O'Brien 1981; Daly 1978; Miller 1976). There is a questioning of the nature of the institution of motherhood (Rich 1976; Arms 1975; Rothman 1982). There is a questioning of the view of child care as the primary responsibility of the mother (Dinnerstein 1977; Chodorow 1978; Ruddick 1983). There is concern with women who, for whatever reason, work outside of the home (Oakley 1980b; Russell and Fitzgibbons 1982). Even the question of whether to have children at all is now open to reflection (Dowrick and Grundberg 1980; Trebilcot 1983). Women are also learning about their own bodies and in so doing are producing an energy that leads to an exploration of all aspects of their lives. "Learning to understand, accept, and be responsible for our physical selves, . . . we can be better friends and better lovers, better *people*, more self-confident, more autonomous, stronger, and more whole" (Boston Women's Health Book Collective 1984: xix).

When women speak, simply as women, about childbearing and mothering, they do so amidst a clamor of other voices: nurses, childbirth educators, medical doctors, sociologists, psychologists, and other scholars. What distinguishes these women's voices from the experts (be they women or men) is that the women tend to speak from their own experiences of how they live in this world as childbearing women and mothers. One has only to review the current popular books about pregnancy and childbirth available to childbearing women (see current ICEA *Bookmarks*), skim the medical and nursing textbooks (Clark and Affonso 1976; Field 1984; Pritchard, Mac-Donald, and Gant 1985), investigate what childbirth educators are teaching (Kitzinger 1979b; Simkin, Whalley, and Keppler 1984), or read recent feminist literature (Firestone 1970; Daly 1978; O'Brien 1981; Oakley 1984; Morgan 1984; Corea 1985) to know that differing opinions about the childbirth experience abound.

There are women who think birth should happen at home; other women feel that the hospital is the place of birth. Some women want minimal use of technological or professional intervention; others accept both without any hesitation. Some want a midwife to support, guide, and help with birthing the baby; others want an obstetrician or a general practitioner to be present at the delivery. Some feel that women should be in control and take the responsibility to make the decisions which affect themselves and their babies; others feel that professionals have the rights and obligations to make the decisions. Some use human satisfaction as a criterion to judge the outcome of childbirth; others cite mortality and morbidity statistics in the evaluation. Some women see childbirth as a disruption in their lives, and other women feel that it is a peak experience which profoundly changes the very core of their being. Some see a need to free women from the shackles of childbirth and mothering; others see the possibility of childbirth as an important celebration of femininity—the very strength of being female.

THE SITUATION

The situation of the childbearing women is a complex one—exemplified by the differing approaches to childbirth knowledge. Two women's stirring descriptions of the birth of their first child exemplify two differing applications of knowledge and opinions. Both Gail and Christine are Canadian women with similar backgrounds and expectations of the childbirth process. Gail's daughter was born in a large, tertiary care hospital in Tanzania. Reflecting on the last moments of labor, she said:

> Then the team gathered around . . . all women [three midwives, two nurses] and they were incredible! There were no stirrups, right! It was all hands-on! Everyone had some part of me. One was holding one leg, one was holding the other leg. I was held by all these women, and I remember only minutes before the last, all of us just laughing. Them joking about something. Just before the last contraction grabbed me, I had to stop myself from this big laugh that I was in. It just seemed that there was just so much gaiety—that only a whole collection of women together like that could really see the humor of that moment. There was something about the magic of that last bit of time. Then she was born. Who would have thought, who can think that actually delivering a baby, painful, well yes, can actually be kind of fun.(G)[1]

Christine described her birthing experience differently. She had been in labor for many hours:

> Then things got really busy, seems to me there were three nurses, and there was another doctor assisting with the birth, and Dr. Henry gave me a pudendal block, and I remember knowing what that was, seeing a picture in the textbook, and that was all right. I was in stirrups and they had put the green things on, and were very busy, and everyone was draping me with stuff. I was thinking about the pudendal block and the nerves it hit. It hurt a bit, not really bad, very quick. And then they gave me a local down towards my anus, and that really hurt, hurt more than anything. I was still not looking at anyone, not looking at Dr. Henry, not seeing the forceps. I know I had my eyes open but I don't remember seeing anyone, and he said, "With the next contraction, I want you to push, I have the forceps on, and I want you to push." I didn't feel him put them on, didn't feel a thing when they were applied. Then Nathan [husband], and the nurses told me, at the same time, that there was a

contraction and I started to push and that was the worst thing I have ever felt in my entire life (laughs). I just felt that everything was being pulled and yanked. The pain was so excruciating, I stopped pushing, and I think everybody . . . Dr. Henry said, "Christine, push," and I can remember him being louder than I had ever heard him. And Nathan said, "Push now," and then what happened was that everything stopped because I stopped pushing. My legs went straight out of my hip (I think I bonked the resident with my foot), my feet went out, and I yelled and yelled and said, "I can't push, it hurts." I must have pushed a little bit more and then Dr. Henry told me I was to "push the baby out on my own." He had taken the forceps off and the baby was born. . . . They finished with a zillion stitches, I'm sure. And then he (the doctor) came to my side and said, "Boy, I don't ever want you to do that to me again,"—that is what he said to me. (C3)

Of course there are a number of aspects which would affect these experiences, such as the position of the baby, the energy of the mother, the length of the labor, the differing cultures, and/or the hospital policy, but what must also be recognized is that implicit in these influences is the application of knowledge.

In the one situation one senses the closeness, the touch of women, who brought their skill, humor, and knowledge to assist the birthing woman to relax and open herself to the birth of her child. Perhaps in their wisdom these carriers of childbirth knowledge intuited the connection between the relaxed, laughing woman and the relaxed and flexible perineal muscles. Their practices showed thoughtful support for Gail to birth her own child. In the other situation one senses the effort made to prevent infection (the green drapes), to prevent pain (by inflicting pain), with the doctors, nurses, and husband using their knowledge and understanding in directing the experience, even to the point of telling Christine when her contractions were occurring (information available through the fetal monitor). The doctor's comment to Christine after the birth, even if said in jest, reveals a sense of whose experience was central. Yet both experiences resulted in the birth of a healthy, living child and mother. So what is at stake? What is the problem? Is there a problem?

When I was a young girl of perhaps twelve or thirteen, I read Pearl Buck's *The Good Earth*. When O-lan, the wife of Wang Lung, said to her husband, "I am with child," I was intrigued. I was drawn back to those descriptions of birth a number of times. This was O-lan's first child.

She would have no one with her when her hour came. . . . She said no word. . . . The panting of the woman became quick and loud, like whispered screams, but she made no sound aloud . . . [then] a thin, fierce cry came. . . . She called him in. The red candle was lit and she was lying neatly covered upon the bed. Beside her, wrapped in a pair of his old trousers, as the custom was in this part, lay his son. (Buck 1931: 37–39)

However mythical this description of non-Western, traditional birth may be, it does give a contrast to present Western practice. In our society, women do not give birth squatting over an old tub they keep for that purpose. They do not creep around the room afterwards to remove traces of the birth, like an animal does. They do not hide the bucket of blood under the bed so no one will see. They do not say with the birth of the girl-child, "It is over once more. It is only a slave this time—not worth mentioning" (p. 62). O-lan gave birth in the tradition of her time. She gave birth as she understood herself and her life. She was a good woman. Childbirth was her responsibility.

In 1974 when pregnant with my second child I decided that I wanted my new baby to stay with me from the moment of birth. Hospital practice at that time separated mothers and babies for a 12–hour observation period.[2] During those hours the baby was kept swaddled in a blanket and placed under a warm light in a clear plastic bassinet. It was in 1972 that Klaus and Kennell's research suggested that extended contact between the baby and mother at birth assists in better mothering. This research demonstrated the importance of the first postpartum hours and days for the development of maternal attachment. Unfortunately for me, this research had not yet reached northern Canada. I knew that it would be necessary for me to have "scientific" research to support my request, so I armed myself with this latest research, including animal studies, and anything else I could glean from libraries to prepare myself to face my obstetrician and the head nurse of the maternity ward. Although both reminded me of how tired I would be, and that new babies need constant care, with one even declaring that babies "like" to be in the nursery, it was agreed that—given a healthy child and an uncomplicated birth—my baby could stay by my side. My daughter was born late one Saturday afternoon into the hands of the doctor who arrived just in time to put on sterile gloves and who left two or three minutes later. The head nurse did not work on weekends, and the agreement posted on the bulletin board in the nursing station was not sufficiently powerful to change routine. So I was left standing outside the nursery window looking at my new child.

My experience illustrates a number of points. First, childbirth practices change over time, depending on the current research available or on who is in charge (Green 1985). Now mothers and fathers are encouraged to stay with their child for at least one hour or more after delivery (Klaus and Kennell 1976; Young 1978). If women are too exhausted or otherwise unable to attend their child at this time, it is noted on the chart as an incident of concern to staff (Field 1984: 79). Secondly, scientific knowledge or opinion is more powerful than personal knowledge or opinion. There is, however, a beginning realization that the "scientific" model of research appropriate for the natural sciences, is not necessarily the best form of research for understanding the human situation, and health care in particular (Buytendijk 1974; Polanyi 1969; Pelletier 1979; Bergsma and Thomasma 1982; Cousins 1983). Research that attempts to understand the way experiences are lived by humans is now being introduced in many fields of human science research. The third point is that routine childbirth practices are often carried out for their own sake. Routines such as perineal shaving, enema, episiotomies, or the 12-hour separation are often practiced routinely without the support of scientific research findings or consideration of individual wishes (Stewart and Stewart 1976). There needs to be constant re-evaluation of routines that become engraved into practice. The last and most important point for the current discussion is that knowledge used in childbirth practices affects women's understanding of themselves.

Again let's look back at my experience: I was excited about the birth of another child, and a girl, too. Now we had a boy and a girl. The labor was intense and, at times, overwhelming. I handled it with the support of my husband and nursing staff. I felt good. My separation from my newly born daughter was a disappointment. Yet, I began to think, "Perhaps, they are right after all. The routine is there for a purpose. Perhaps I couldn't handle the situation if she choked and turned blue. What if something did happen to her if she were left in my care? Could something happen to her?" The self-doubts that gradually seeped into my thoughts encouraged me to stand back from what I had previously known as right and good—the importance of being with my child; to let the experts do what in their opinion was right and good—the need to maintain routine and control.

As I think more distantly about that woman at the nursery window, and the baby in the bassinet, I wonder if there is even more at stake here than originally thought. What makes a woman a mother? Does it have to do with watching, holding, nursing, diapering, and even suctioning? Yes, of course, it is all those things. But is it not more, also? But what? How did that mother know something the scientists did not *yet* know? How was her understanding of herself as a mother different from their understanding of mothers? How do approaches to knowledge used in childbirth contribute to the understanding a woman attains as she becomes a mother? Gail and Christine gave birth under the influence of the present traditions of childbirth knowledge. It is true that their experiences are just individual instances making generalization impossible. That is, however, not the point. The point is, rather, to show the need to analyze what *is* at stake.

The effort to assist women to make knowledgeable decisions from a menu of possible choices, many of them "hard choices" (Colen 1986), has been an important endeavor of childbirth educators, childbirth education associations, ethics committees, and scholars. The first concern is the health of the mother and baby, and, secondly, the emotional fulfillment of the mother, father, and family (as if they are separable!). It is recognized that for most people, "becoming parents [mothers] is a greater life change than any other they will experience" (Simkin et al. 1984: 3).

How does a woman "live" childbirth knowledge? It is from this situation that the focus of this book becomes intelligible. The primary question is, therefore: "How does a woman come to understand herself as mother?" or stated differently: "How does the experience of childbirth transform woman to mother?" *What is the nature of the transformation of woman to mother?*

THE TALK OF WOMEN

> The subject of birth has, inevitably, its own compelling attraction. No one who has given birth or witnessed it ever quite forgets. Mothers relive it secretly, or reflect on their own experience among each other for many years afterwards. For a story that is, essentially, always the same . . . the essence is always new, always dramatic. . . . It was the same for Cleopatra, for Marie de Medici, for Anna Magdelena Bach and Sophia Tolstoy and Sophia Loren and—Eve. I was in good company. (Sorel 1984: xvi)

Women tell each other about their childbirth experiences. They reminisce about labor and delivery. They talk about feelings—what made them feel good —when they felt bad. This talk occurs around kitchen tables, at baby showers, at bus stops, over cups of tea, almost anywhere there are pregnant women and mothers. In spite of the fact that almost all births are normal, that is, without medical complications, it is often the horror stories of labor and delivery that are told. "I am afraid 'cause everyone tells me all those stories about when you have your first baby, you are in labor for hours, and hours, and hours, and hours," said a young pregnant woman. Brenda said, "I find a lot of people will tell me horror stories. They always tell me the worst, the bad things that can happen. I just take them with a grain of salt. I have to take this in my stride" (B1). Why does the talk often focus on the pain or hardship? Is it for dramatic effect? Is it because women really have had such a bad time?

Through talking together, many woman have come to realize that they may have missed an important event of their lives as women. Women who were unconscious, sedated, or delivered by cesarean sections have also begun to question their experiences. Others, like Christine, say, "I'm glad I didn't miss it—the pain—the work. It was something I did not want to miss" (C1). A few years ago a newspaper columnist wrote a series of articles tracing the change in birthing practices over the last thirty years (Sweet 1983). Many women, in response to the series, wrote or telephoned the paper with stories that were traumatic, "heart-breaking," according to the columnist. Through sharing their own stories, women have begun to realize that their individual unsatisfactory experiences were not just personal failures but were experiences that were shared by others (Jordan 1980: 86). "Who among us has not been dumbfounded at the realization that those problems so modestly brought up [in conversations] were the lot of almost all women" (Fauré 1981: 83)? Women's changing consciousness, revealing the dark side of their common experiences of childbirth, has brought about change, such as universal childbirth education classes, the routine presence of fathers in the delivery room, the return of the midwife, and other humanizing practices. Phyllis Chesler wrote, "There's a shelf in my local bookstore marked 'Child Care,' with books by male experts on annual expected growth rates and separation anxiety; books praising natural childbirth; books damning obstetrical practices in America. . . . I find [only] a handful of precious, brave books, all published in the last five years, by mothers on motherhood" (1979: 4). The stories of women, by women, are beginning to surface. Thus, instead of shrinking women's experience of birth into clinical terms or breaking it into fragments through much of present day research, the talk of women is directed toward the construction of new understanding of experiences true to the reality of their lives.

Women's talk has real value, for talk is the very vehicle for change—for re-creation of the world in their own voice (Berger and Luckmann 1967; Gilligan 1982). Some women talk and write about childbirth for their own personal reflection, while more and more are writing to share with others (Chicago 1985; Barrington 1985: chap. 7; Ashford 1984; Sorel 1984; Dowrick and Grundberg 1980; Kitzinger 1978). Many women want to know about childbirth and mothering, especially those women who are pregnant. They "search for Mothers, dead and alive, to guide them," said Chesler (1979: 5). Judy Chicago in describing her work of the *Birth Project* talked about meetings where women speak about their birth experiences. "It was spellbinding and very moving. It made me wonder why there has been so little art about birth" (1985: 19). Childbirth is an important life event, an experience that needs to be uncovered or, perhaps, recovered by women themselves.

Becoming a mother is an inner journey for women. Of course, it is an outer one too—marked by the burgeoning waist, the ballooning clothes, the awkward gait, and, for many, a radiant and wholesome face. The integrated reality of both the outer and the inner process is traced in this book through listening to and talking with women who are in the midst of their own experiences of becoming mothers. O'Brien (1981: 8) argued that it is "from an adequate understanding of the process of reproduction, nature's traditional and bitter trap for the suppression of women, that women can begin to understand their possibilities and their freedom." This book is intended to broaden that understanding.

RESEARCHING WOMEN'S EXPERIENCE

To begin to understand the process of reproduction, how it changes woman to mother, we need to explore the lives of women through their talk about their own lives, instead of decontextualizing women's experiences which loses the meaning we need to capture. To search for "understanding" of women's experience rather than "explanation," (in the narrower scientific or empirical-analytic sense), I use a phenomenological approach—of which hermeneutics or interpretation is an integral aspect.

Stated in a simple way, phenomenology has to do with description of experience and hermeneutics with interpretation. Such simplicity, however, contradicts the depth and complexity of the historical roots from which these philosophical approaches arise. Phenomenology is associated especially with the foundational writings of philosophers such as Edmund Husserl (1970, 1977), Martin Heidegger (1962, 1971, 1977a), and Maurice Merleau-Ponty (1962, 1964, 1968). Others have infused the phenomenological project with a concern for hermeneutics (Gadamer 1975; Ricoeur 1973), a concern for a hermeneutical epistemology (Rorty 1979), power (Foucault 1975, 1978, 1983), critical theory (Habermas 1968), textuality, (Derrida 1973), and so forth. Most, if not all, of these approaches are fundamentally concerned with understanding the lived meaning of the life world—an interpretation of human experience.

> Phenomenological research edifies the depthful, the personal insight contributing to one's thoughtfulness and one's ability to act toward others, child or adults, with a tact or tactfulness. . . . We might say that phenomenology is a philosophy of the unique, the personal, the individual which we pursue, against the background of an understanding of the logos of Other, the Whole, or the Communal. (van Manen 1984a: ii)

The hermeneutic phenomenological approach of this work (based on the work of van Manen) uses both description, which is concerned with the lived experience of women in childbirth, and hermeneutics, which is the act of interpretation, as a way to recover the nature of lived experience of women becoming mothers.

When we talk about "lived experience" we talk about the experience of being in the world, the world of everyday life, the world as it is experienced.

> Lived experience is the "originary" way in which we perceive reality. As living persons we have an awareness of things and ourselves which is immediate, direct, and nonabstractive. We "live through" (*erleben*) life with an intimate sense of its concrete, qualitative features and myriad patterns, meanings, values, and relations. (Ermarth 1978: 97)

To speak of our lived experience in a strong sense is to go beyond the taken-for-granted. It is to "uncover meanings in everyday practice in such a way that they are not destroyed, distorted, decontextualized, trivialized or sentimentalized" (Benner 1985:6). It is to explore the way in which pregnant, childbearing, and mothering women experience the world. It is an intensified exploration of women's own realities—the shape of their own lived worlds (Greene 1978). This exploration centers around ongoing conversation with women. It is a search for understanding of women who express themselves through their talk.

Conversations

In order to explore the experience of transformation as lived by women in childbirth, I engaged in conversations with women before, during, and after pregnancy and birth. These conversations were of two distinct types, the one-time conversation, and the in-depth series of conversations. Women generally want to talk about their birth experiences. Over the years of my study I have conversed with many mothers. Others I met said, "I'd like to talk to you—I have something to tell." I was also influenced by my presence at the home birth of a friend (P1).

With some women, for example, the conversations were for investigating specific experiences, such as the use of the fetal monitor, or the experience of birthing pain, while six women were followed intensively from mid-pregnancy to a number of months of living with the child. These six women were all first-time mothers. Brenda and Susan were brought into the study through contact with their obstetricians, Anna and Katherine were approached through the midwife who planned to attend their home births, and Christine and Jane were recruited through friends and associates. Because these women were comparable in age, background, and financial status, one might notice a similarity in their language and the nature of their talk. As urban Canadians they offer a particular view of their experience of becoming mothers.

The term "conversation" rather than "interview" is chosen to describe the actual process that was used. With each woman I talked about the nature of my interest in exploring women's experience of childbirth (including pregnancy and postpartum). As they agreed to continue the conversation, they signed a consent form which indicated their willingness to participate. It was understood that they could withdraw from the study whenever they wished. None did. I encouraged all of them to talk about how it was for them and to use concrete events as anecdotal examples. The following questions are examples of the ways I initiated or prompted conversations with the six women who became the main focus of the study:

When did the possibility of children first come up? or did it?
What kinds of feelings did you have when you found out for sure that you were pregnant?
How did others in your life respond?
What was your experience of body, space, time? Did you find yourself seeing, hearing things, or attending to things you did not before?
What are the days like? At what times or moments are you reminded of your pregnancy? or the child inside you? What is it like? How do you feel?
Do you think ahead sometimes? What occurs to you?
Do you think about the birth? In what way? How do you feel about that?

The atmosphere of the conversation was open and an effort was made to have the women speak with as much specificity as possible about their own experience in order to clarify what they meant. "Can you give me an example?" was often my only interjection into their talk. (Phenomenological research has been called the "science of examples.")

My relationship with the women was friendly and enjoyable. With each I sensed a feeling of mutual respect and openness. The women participated in the study for their own reasons. Perhaps it was curiosity; perhaps they saw it as an opportunity to talk to an interested person about their own experiences; perhaps they thought they might learn something; or perhaps they wanted to contribute to research in this area. For whatever reasons the women participated, they gave generously of their time, and more importantly, of their experiences, thoughts, and feelings. They allowed me to "touch" their inner experience of transformation as well as to discuss their outward reactions and perceptions of what was taking place in their lives.

One woman, Brenda, and her husband, agreed to my request to attend the birth of their child which took place in a local hospital. Two of the women's husbands shared in some of the conversations, and over a period of time I had the opportunity to meet all the men. Although my primary interest is in women's experiences, the women's involvement with their partners was an important element that ran through much of their talk. All the women seemed to have strong and committed relationships during this period of time. All but two of the ongoing conversations took place in the women's homes. The two exceptions took place in the privacy of Christine's office. Brief hospital visits were made when possible, and the first postpartum conversation was held as soon as possible following the birth. All the conversations were recorded on audio tape and transcribed. Considerable disruption occurred during the conversations that took place following the births, demonstrating vividly the changed character of the women's lives.

Conversations with only six women may seem to give a limited view of experience. However, each conversation offered a rich and deep wealth of material that demands even more extensive exploration than is offered here. I do not expect that this analysis is a conclusive or final commentary on women's transformative experiences of childbirth and becoming mothers. It is offered as one possible interpretation in the effort to strive for a deeper understanding of women's lives.

I was conscious of the interaction between each woman and myself during these conversations. The women were experiencing the birth of a first child; I have two children now thirteen and fifteen years old. The women were in their late 20s or early 30s; I am over forty. Their everyday lives were filled with work and home; mine with study of their experience, along with an intensive dwelling in the literature of women, childbirth, and phenomenology. I was very interested in their experience, they were not exploring mine. But I was not merely a privileged observer—I was involved. At the same time as there was a sharing of a common concern and experience, the mutuality was inevitably skewed by the research intentions. But still, as we talked together, aspects of our lives were present—in the "in-between"—we came to the conversations as people (Gadamer 1975).

In delineating the "in-between," it must be understood that in conversations of this nature both participants are immersed in the tradition of their own life history. It is from this position of shared history that understanding comes into being. At the same time, there needs to be full consciousness of the presuppositions and interests that are carried, and there needs to be a recognition that these "common-sense preunderstandings, suppositions, assumptions, and the existing bodies of scientific knowledge predispose us to interpret the nature of the phenomenon before we have even come to grips with the significance of the phenomenological questions" (van Manen 1984a: 9). Therefore instead of "bracketing," that is, setting aside certain questions and assumptions, I attempted to question the "taken for grantedness," to look at what is truly being said in the conversation. Such questioning allows for new understandings, new possibilities, that may go beyond the reality of the presuppositions. It demands a critical consciousness on my part to acknowledge and attend to my own presuppositions so as to arrive at the depth of the phenomenon (Kvale 1984).

Stories

Knowledge has been lost in the surge toward "research data" and "information," which to be considered valid must be objective, factual, and replicable. Stories, in contrast, are contextualized, personal knowledge, never replicable, and full of life experience which is not explained. Thus, with stories, nothing is forced on the reader, as with interpretation or analysis. The reader can enter the story in a manner that ties the reader to the story in a personal way. Benjamin says that the loss of storytelling as a valued enterprise is related to the changed "face of death" in present society. He contends that people are "dry dwellers in eternity" who at their end are stowed away in sanatoriums or hospitals (1969: 94). While once the death of a person could release the story of personal knowledge and wisdom—"the stuff of real life"—the hygienic approach to death has led to a loss of the authority of storytelling.

The story, however, offers a way to approach human experience. From the conversations with the six women the stories were developed. Each woman's story is unique with its own rhythm. Its authority is perceived by the readers as they interpret from their own experience. In Chapter 2 I take excerpts from the transcripts and reconstruct each woman's story to reflect what stood out in her talk and seemed central to her life. I do this by thinking about each woman and asking myself what is the nature of her talk. What are her interests and concerns? How does she show herself to me? Presented in this way, the stories introduce each woman and tell her story in a way that reveals the landscape of her life—her situation and the context from which her words came. With understanding and respect for the complexity of these women's lives, and all human life, the story that characterizes a particular woman's life is, naturally, a simplification of that life.

While the writing of the stories comes out of my reflection on our conversations (that is, there is choice in the telling), the words belong to each woman. Nothing is fictionalized. The women were invited to read and comment on their story as it is presented. Each agreed that she was able to see aspects of her experience in the story. On the one hand, it is to be acknowledged that as a story captures only a few aspects of a particular woman's life, it may be less truly her personal story but another version of Woman. On the other hand, the retelling, the interpreting, the focusing, and the shaping may make for a different and, in some sense, a better understanding of a woman's life.

Thematic Moments

As I read the stories I began to notice that each somehow characterized a particular theme. It was as if the themes, or thematic moments, came out of the stories themselves—they "showed themselves," in a sense, as they were discovered after the stories were written. Moreover, in reflecting on each woman's uniqueness and what stood out of her individual story, it became apparent that these moments were found in the other women's stories as well. It would have been easy to create dialogue among the women themselves on these overlapping moments. The use of the word "moments" instead of the word "themes" seems to capture in a better way the special aspects that are highlighted through these stories. These moments are not periods of time, although they occur over time, but are identifiable aspects of this experience that interact together to show the change from woman to mother.

It is important not to make too much of thematic moments. For example, while it is true that coming to a decision about having a child is part of all women's move to motherhood, yet, for each woman, the decision may be experienced differently or may not be dealt with thoughtfully (Chapter 3). Consider, too, the theme of responsibility (Chapter 6). Responsibility is an important aspect of the move to motherhood, but it may be realized in different ways and at different times by individual women. It is also true that there may be other moments that could be found, such as the woman's changing relationship with her mother, or the changed recognition of the importance of grandparents. Thematic moments should rather be seen as "knots in the webs of our experiences, around which lived experiences are spun, and are experienced as meaningful wholes" (van Manen 1984a: 29). Thus thematic moments are not magically appearing essences, but are useful focal points, or commonalities, of experience, around which phenomenological interpretation can occur.

There is a great contrast between the story and its interpretation. The thematic moments presented in Chapters 3 to 7 represent further interpretive work with the texts of the transcripts by: tracing etymological sources, searching idiomatic phrases, exploring other childbirth literature and artistic sources, and attending to personal experience (van Manen 1984a). Through thematic analysis I explore the women's words to discover the forgotten, hidden, mysterious, or ambiguous nature of their experiences. These dimensions of meaning a person cannot easily discover by herself or himself. It is a hermeneutic project—an interaction with the various materials (texts)— that discloses meanings. The possibility of phenomenological interpretation is to produce or establish meaning by exploring the situation, the choices, and the actions that describe the meaning context of experience.

> The stress is not upon the subjective interests of the interpreter nor upon the objective features of the work itself, but on the art of interpreting and the significance of the interpretation that is produced. Phenomenological description is an account of the meaning of something, phenomenological interpretation is the *act* of producing or establishing a meaning. (Silverman 1984: 22)

Through the dialectic going back and forth among the various levels of questioning there is a striving for a thoughtfulness, "a deeply reflective activity that involves the totality of our physical and mental being" (van Manen 1984a: 28). In one sense, it is an exploration of self, forcing a self-reflective attitude. I have been forced to attend to the question of "Who am I?" as a woman and as a mother.

The Writing

Phenomenological writing is integral to this research approach. The writing, as interpretation, strives for a poetic (disclosing) quality in that it attempts to bring to language the thematic moments in such a way that the essence, or the lived-through meaning of the experience shows itself.

To organize the writing, the existential themes of temporality (lived time), spatiality (lived space), corporeality (lived body), and communality (lived relationship to others) have been woven into the thematic moments revealed by the women's stories. Along with this visual structuring of the writing, the effort was made to search for deeper levels of analysis, to vary examples, and to explore and engage in a dialogical fashion with other texts. It is immersion in language, the shared meanings, that makes the interpretive process possible. Language both reveals and conceals—providing for a unity between the said and the unsaid (Gadamer 1975). "More is meant than intended in each expression, and thus the hermeneutic process is needed to explicate the unsaid" (Idhe 1983: 151). It is a project that moves from life towards thoughts, not backwards to the author, but forward to its meaning and toward the sort of world it discovers and opens up (Marcel 1978; Ricoeur 1973).

Habermas (1968) outlined three types of knowledge arising from particular interests—an interest in understanding, technical interest, and emancipatory interest. The interest of this study has been in understanding—yet the underlying concern has been emancipatory. The possibility of getting beyond the surface level of the phenomenon, to the deeper than conventional wisdom, implies a critical stance. It has action potential, suggested by the questions: "How do we create a world that supports and encourages women with children to live as mothers?" "How does the woman come to know herself as mother in our present health care environment?" "What does it mean to be a health care professional in the midst of women's transformative experiences?" The emancipatory, critical aspect is inherent in the entire work.

Limitations

As I complete this research I am aware of its possibilities as well as its limitations. How are the possibilities of this research going to make a difference to the company of women who give birth—daughters who become mothers in the future? Some of the limitations are implicit in the method and may easily be identified, while others are more problematic as they are not so easily seen. In this study, there was no expectation that results would be arrived at which would be generalizable to all women who become mothers, that the study would be able to be replicated to yield the same data, or that a description of a transformative experience could be understood in such a way as to lead to measurement or even to comparisons between women's transformative experiences. Research into matters profoundly human, as attempted here, cannot be generalizable, reductionist, or measurable. In order to evaluate and extend this work, a study using a similar approach, in conversation with younger women, for example, or with women from other cultures, would provide the opportunity to come to a deeper understanding of women's transformative experiences of becoming mothers.

The more problematic limitations of this study may well be found in other directions. Parse, Coyne, and Smith (1985) suggested standards used to guide evaluation appraisal: the soundness of ideas (supported by appropriate evidence), the presentation of ideas (organized in a succinct way with clarity and integration), the attention given to the self-determination of the participants, and clear explanation of the methodological and interpretive dimensions. Yet as I consider how soundness of ideas is evaluated, I recognize that with this work the soundness of the ideas may not be seen until the work is brought into discussion with others.

The limitations were brought to test as I gave Chapters 3 to 8 to Susan, Anna, Christine, and Katherine for their comments. I felt vulnerable and reluctant to present an analysis of their conversations. Each woman carefully read the work and commented through writing and discussion. Two of the conversations lasted almost two hours as we explored, clarified, and expanded the various ideas. It would have been worthwhile to have had all the women discuss the work together. Susan and Christine offered these written comments:

What I found most interesting was discovering that the other women in the study had many similar feelings and experiences as I did—feeling the vulnerability, a change in treatment by others, and even something as trivial as lack of choice of clothing. . . . All of us had made the decision to have children and then having conceived were struck by the over-whelming feelings of uncertainty. It was reassuring to know other women felt the same. (S7)

It was indeed a transformation for me. . . . I was interested in those things that seemed common (the inwardness one feels during labor), and how we differed (how we felt about our changing bodies). There is great strength derived from birthing and mothering and I think it is an untapped resource. (C8)

It may be that the limitations of research such as this will only be fully comprehended through continued conversations that explore the data with the courage to rethink, discard, clarify, expand, and deepen the ideas presented here. Such conversations, begun in the company of women, need to include partners, friends, practitioners, researchers, and scholars who strive to understand this important experience in women's lives.

Chapter 2

Gathering Fragments of Women's Experience

There are women everywhere with fragments
    gather fragments
    weave and mend
When we learn to come together we are whole.
                   —Anne Cameron

THE STORIES

By gathering the fragments and threads from the stories of women it may be possible to weave a fabric that displays the transformation of women who become mothers. Each story, with its own texture, its own feeling, its own image, arises from incidents in the everyday lives of these women. Each story reaches below the surface uncovering fragments of one person's experience which others can incorporate (Kotre 1984). Storytelling, as an interpersonal event, carries with it traces of the storyteller clinging to the text—like the hand prints of the potter on the clay vessel (Benjamin 1969). In this way it is different from journals, diaries, memoirs, or autobiographies (Kotre 1984). Here, then, are the stories of Brenda, Christine, Jane, Susan, Anna, and Katherine.

Brenda

Brenda and Tom live in a new city development, the houses spaced "inches" apart. Two large dogs meet me at the door as I visit for the first time. Brenda is twenty-six. She has always thought they would have a child sooner or later.

"We have been married five years this December and we decided that we have our house, have our dogs, have our vehicles, so it is more or less time. Actually I wanted to wait another year, but I will be twenty-seven next week and if we want two children, I'd better get started. Tom really did not want to wait, so I agreed to have the IUD taken out with the hope that it would take a few months to get pregnant.

"But two weeks later I never got my period and I was shocked. I was shocked and I cried. Tom laughed because he was so happy, ecstatic. Just like a little kid. He had wanted children for so long.

"I said, 'No, Tom, this can't happen that fast, no way.' But of course, I was. The first reaction was upset. I thought, 'How could it happen so fast, here I am going to be a mom and I don't want to be a mom just like that.' Thank God it takes five or six months before you really start to show.

"It was just shocking. I spent the whole summer being sick. Morning sickness. At work, with all the heavy lifting, I'd get cramps. And the sun. It was such a beautiful summer. I would go outside for five minutes, and I would be upstairs in the bathroom again. Or we would go camping and I'd be sick the whole time, from the time I got up until the time I went to bed. It went on all of June and July. It was near the end of August I started to feel better. In a way you could say I was talked into getting pregnant. But I'm not sorry now, but at the time I was. 'Tom, how could you do this to me!' That kind of thing.

"At work, people drive me crazy. It's, 'Mom this, and Mom that.' Just to get used to people coming up and wanting to touch your belly, like there must be a hundred staff in that store, and they are so thrilled to see a pregnant person, and they come up and want to feel your baby kicking. It really embarrasses me. But what do you say? 'I don't want you feeling my baby.' Like it is too personal, and they want to know everything. Like, 'Were you sick this morning?' and 'Did you drive to work?' It gets to the point, 'Leave me alone, I am only pregnant, not a baby!'

"In a lot of ways the baby comes first for other people. They say, 'Brenda, you shouldn't be doing that.' 'Your hands shouldn't be over your head, you shouldn't lift that.' 'Yes dear,' I say, mocking them. 'Yes, I won't do that anymore, I'm sorry, I was a bad girl,' and then I would turn around and do it.

"And I've noticed that you go into a crowded place, and a lot of people look at you and smile. Whereas before you could just walk in. When you go to a place, like Saturday night we went for a drink in a lounge, and I find that people really make you feel uneasy, like you are doing something just terrible, and you are only drinking orange juice. Like 'come on!'

"I want to go back to work. I get so bored if I have two days off in a row. I like to get out and do something. I don't like to be stuck at home. But maybe with a child, you would be doing things. We have a lady next door who will babysit. I'll start going back in the evenings and Tom will babysit. But like he says, 'I don't want to sit in the house every Saturday and babysit.' It is the same for me, I don't want to feel that I have to do everything with the baby. I want to have my own life too. If I want to go out with the girls, I should be able to.

"I am going to bottle feed. That was a major fight. Tom believes in mother's milk. And me, just being the type of person I am, I just have an aversion to it. Even if I see someone else nursing it kind of gives me the creepy-crawlies. It is a natural thing and I know it is good for the child and I've heard all the good points about it. But it is just not for me. It's good old formula. Thank goodness they have invented those things.

"Our best friends have a three-month-old boy, and like I have yet to pick it up or anything like that. I am not the type that wants to cuddle or hold it, but they say it is different when it is your own. We will wait and see.

"I would rather have a boy, I don't think I want a girl, mainly because Tom would be too strict with her. I am sure if we had a little girl and she was out playing for two hours, and he didn't see her, it would be like twenty questions. 'Where were you?' 'What house were you in?' 'Who were you playing with?' He wouldn't do that with boys. He does it with me too. Like we will go into a restaurant, and I will ask for something, and he will say, 'No, she doesn't want that, she is pregnant, she is having this.' I get this stunned look on my face and when the waitress leaves, I say,

'Tom, do you realize what you did?'

'No.'

'Tom, I asked for coffee and they are bringing me milk. I don't want milk.'

He feels embarrassed, but I don't think he would notice he was doing it to a girl. Anyway I think it is going to be a boy. We would be happy either way, but I have always felt that we are going to have boys. We have two girl dogs, and will have two boy kids.

"I find it, my body, really hard to accept. You understand that this is a baby growing inside you, and you have to get bigger, and you see your body growing different, and there are deposits of fat and stuff. It disgusts me. So far it is hard, it's firm, but you know that it will be jelly-like later on. It is hard to accept. I step on the scales, and I say, 'I weigh that much?' I believe that you can have a child and you can go back down to 115 pounds afterwards, there is no reason why you shouldn't. I feel that I should be the way I was before.

"We saw a film about natural childbirth and cesarean section at the prenatal class. I kept my eyes closed. 'Just let me know when it is over.' Tom was really impressed. Now he wants me to have a cesarean. He says it is more humane, like he doesn't like to see a woman suffer. He figures it would be less pain. I think it would be harder on your whole body with getting used to the baby and not feeling as well as you could. I don't want it, but I don't think I will have any choice in the matter. Whatever is going to be is going to be."

Later, at the hospital . . .

Brenda was moved to the delivery room and when asked how she was feeling said, "I don't know. I just want to get this over with."

Everything was happening so fast. The doctor came in, gowned, and put Brenda's feet in the stirrups. Although Brenda mentioned the cramp in her leg, there was no attention paid to it; there was no time to attempt to relieve the cramp. The doctor said that on the next contraction the baby would be born. He cut an episiotomy, and the baby slipped out. The baby responded quickly and cried.

"It's a girl!" said the doctor.

"No!"

"I am going to put the baby on your stomach."

"No, please don't."

The doctor then held the baby until the cord was clamped, which was almost right away, and gave the baby to the midwife who wrapped it and put it under the lights in the bassinet. Brenda commented about having a flat stomach and smiled when she talked of it. From the end of the room, the midwife involved herself with records and procedures. The doctor repaired the episiotomy and the obstetrician again asked if Brenda would like to hold her baby. "No." Her head was turned away from the baby.

In masks covering our noses and mouths, Tom and I stood and looked at the baby. She was beautiful. I wanted to hold her, and suggested to Tom that he might. Neither of us did.

Christine

"We had ten years together without another person with us," Christine pointed out over a cup of coffee. We sat at the wooden kitchen table that, I guess, she and Nathan had built together. Her home showed care and effort: the stained glass in the front window caught my attention as I arrived.

Christine talked of her life with Nathan. "We always have lots to come home with, we talk about our various jobs, we know a lot about each other's work, and we can ask each other's opinion about this or that problem to which we can comment knowledgeably because we are close enough to know what goes on," she said.

At home, also, their work was shared. When they bring lumber and supplies for the various projects they, together, haul the stuff into the house. Generally Nathan does the constructing and Christine sands and stains. She said, "We have been very equal partners in sharing, both in the household chores and income and in our expectations of working together for certain goals, financial or otherwise." The money they shared was their money, not his, or hers, but from a common pot.

What would bringing another being into their life do to this shared adventure? Christine wondered. What would it mean to them?

Christine was thirty-two. She wanted to make a decision about whether or not to have a baby. Up until she was thirty her focus had been on her career. She desired to do her *own* work, to fulfill ambitions, and yet the possibility of a child in her life kept coming up. She did not want to turn thirty-six or thirty-seven and feel that the decision had been made for her, that she had missed the time for children. In her need to make a decision, she began to pressure Nathan. He did not like that very much. "It puts your relationship in jeopardy," said Christine. "Could having a baby be the biggest mistake of your life, as Nathan thought? Could it really smash everything?" "Whether or not to have a child" gave them some "heavy-duty" times for some months, with Christine crying and Nathan "up-tight." So they decided to find a third person, a counselor, to "mediate the decision."

"What made this decision so tough?" I wondered. "I've seen women in my work," said Christine, "who look like they have been gobbled up by children and a household and a husband. These women are trying to be very good mothers, and spend a lot of energy doing that. They look after their husband and their children and are responsible for keeping the family together. I've seen women who have lost themselves, in a sense. Everything is for their children, or somebody else, and not them, whether they have a career or not." She talked about the plight of forty-five-to-fifty-year-old women who, after the children have left home, are lost. They do not know how to do simple things that most people cope with in their daily lives.

Christine gave an example of a bright woman who held a top role in government. This woman had done such amazing things. Christine wondered, "Would she be there if she had children? Is it possible to do both? And yet, some women manage all kinds of quite exciting things, and still have a household and children and the whole thing." Christine puzzled, "Will I lose myself in becoming a mother?"

Christine described her pregnant friend who went to the bank to get a loan. This friend had said, "I think it was hard for the bank manager to talk to me. He seemed quite anxious that I was pregnant, 'If I was sitting comfortably,' or 'If everything was all right.' And I was there to get my $5500 loan! They don't treat you like any other person, with questions about your employment, your salary, and so on." This furthers Christine's puzzlement, "Why, if you are with child before or after birth, are you not still a woman?"

Looking after a child may be overwhelming. "I keep thinking," said Christine, "I might be too tired, too bogged down with a zillion diapers and maybe a crying baby, and all the millions and millions of tasks involved with a baby." She elaborated, "You see, work is manageable, you know what you can do, you can have it organized, and you know that you have done this for ten years. Nathan thinks I might get bored at home and wonders what I will do with my time, and I'm just bowled over with the thought of it. I just hope I would be able to make it over the first few months."

And then, what will change in herself? "I wonder about the dependency. . . . It is not something I would want, and I know Nathan would not want. It is because it is an unknown and you have nothing to compare it to, nothing! I think it will make a difference in my life, but still at the back of your mind I question that change. We know there will be change but we can't anticipate making it. It diverges the course of your life forever, and that is not necessarily bad or good, just that men never have to truly deal with that, ever."

Nathan talked to the counselor first—by himself. "The guy sure didn't work hard for his money," laughed Christine, "as the issue seemed to dissolve itself." She remembers walking the dog after being through all that, after the decision was made, "Yes, we will go ahead and have a family." Nathan, on the walk, quietly asked, "Well, how do you feel? Aren't you still afraid?" She was.

Christine was visiting her family in the East when she realized she was pregnant. She waited to tell Nathan when he arrived. They were swimming with the family when Christine went up to the cottage. She called Nathan. "I'm pregnant," she said, "but don't hold your breath. I'm bleeding." Nathan was very shocked and said, "What shall I do, what shall I do?" Christine said, "Nothing, just let me stay here. You go down to my friends and carry on." She was very upset and thought, "After finally making the decision, now what if I can't have kids?"

Jane

From the first talk Jane hinted at the possibility of some change coming in herself as she moved along in pregnancy. She said, "I never really liked kids. I remember talking to my sister-in-law about whether or not we could be mothers because we are not all that gung-ho on children, but everyone assures me that you will like your own, that it will be all right. We kind of questioned whether it was true."

Jane was ambivalent throughout her pregnancy. At six months she said, "There are still times when I am not sure that I want to be a mother. It is a little late now," she goes on with a laugh, "but there are still times when I do not want to give up the freedom. And I'm thoroughly enjoying my job that I have now. And I am afraid it is going to change our relationship. We have had such a good year, such fun. I really don't want our relationship to change."

Both Jane and Jim talked about friends whose relationship had deteriorated, they thought, with the coming of a child. These parents doted on their boy, talked of nothing else, laughing at his antics—"which even," much to Jane's disgust, "included grinding cheerios into the rug!" And about those couples who let their child rule their lives, controlling when they would come to dinner or have a night out! Even on the way to the hospital, in intense labor, Jane expressed doubts about their decision, "I just don't know if we are doing the right thing."

But a year later she said she would like to have four children, "with no hesitation at all!" "I was afraid children were really going to change our lifestyle so that it would be a problem for Jim and I and our relationship. But it hasn't, it's grown in a lot of ways. We both enjoy her so much."

I wondered how this dramatic change had happened.

Early in her pregnancy Jane noticed that she saw pregnant women, and mothers and babies, more. "We (she and Jim) both have noticed babies a lot more than we did before," she said. "We notice pregnant women more, watch them, watch what they do, if they are smoking, or drinking, how big they are. The other day Jim and I were at a restaurant, and Jim was telling me what a great day he had had. I was watching these two kids from two different tables playing shy and watching each other, and was not paying any attention to Jim. He looked around,

'What are you looking at?'
'Those two little kids.'
'You've never paid any attention to kids before.'

"And he is right, I hadn't. But I want to know how parents react to their children and how parenting differs. I don't know anything about parenting, I've never taken a course in it, and nobody offers one. It is a very, very, scary thing, a very big thing. In a lot of ways, it is probably the most important thing you do in your life. We are just supposed to pick it up, and I don't know if I can just pick it up. But we both have had very good parenting, so that should help."

Jim reminded Jane of the time she came home from work and had cried for what seemed like two hours or more after seeing a baby that Jane thought was neglected. Jane explained, "This father came in—it must have been one of those really cold days in December—and this baby must have been, uh, only weeks old. The father came in with the baby wrapped in a thin blanket.

The baby, covered with guck, had crocodile tears running down her face and the father was doing nothing to comfort her. I took the baby, which I would never do in my life, because I don't like kids and I don't like dirty kids. But I held the baby and gave her a soother and she was as good as gold. Later the mother came in and seemed very annoyed that I had her child, and she took it and laid it in her lap and ignored it again. I felt so sorry. I was really moved by that, really upset."

Later, eight months pregnant, Jane said, "Um, I'm not so ambivalent now. The baby kicks and I can see the little appendages sticking out, and that makes a difference. It is alive. It is a real thing. I am still apprehensive but not as ambivalent."

We were sitting in her living room admiring her beautiful baby carriage. "At first I kept staring at it," she remarked, "it is the same size to me now as my carriage was when I played dolls. So the carriage feels like I'm sort of playing house. But then I realize, of course, this is the real thing, the bigger deal. Then the furniture becomes foreign. 'What am I going to do with this stuff and all the clothes that various people are making?' They would fit a doll." Jane told about visiting her sister-in-law and new baby the day after the birth. "We saw this little baby, and it was tiny, tiny, ever so small. I wondered how I could relate to such a little person who didn't smile, wanted just to eat and sleep all the time. No one prepares you for that. It is a lot easier to carry it on the inside."

After Lisa's birth Jane said, "I do a lot more giving than I did before, I have to because Lisa is so much more dependent than a husband ever is. So that changes my perceptions of myself. It also makes me feel pretty good that I can provide for her. I don't think I have lost anything. I can go back to being the person I was after Lisa's grown up or after she's gone to school. I can go back to working and making money and being a provider when she is older. But I can never go back to the time when she's young, and I really enjoy it. The whole nursing issue really struck me. She started eating solids at six months, so that meant that I was totally supporting her life for 15 months. And that really made me feel good, that's a real achievement. I don't have to have a paycheck to prove who I am, even though I thought I would."

"Do you talk about Lisa a lot?" I asked. "Yeah, all the time. Jim and I sit and talk about her all the time . . . but she is so fascinating. We find her so, anyway. Jim and I also spend a lot of time talking about our relationship, and how—that is another we were not prepared for—how much time babies take away from your own relationship. We don't have the same time together, the close times. It is not as easy as I thought it was going to be."

Yet six months later Jane said, "Our relationship has always been good. We feel very fortunate. Jim is so understanding. He is feminine in a lot of ways, in the way that he thinks. He cares what I think, very caring and open, and also very patient. With Lisa it's enhanced. We kid about what we're going to do to her, how soon we are going to have to "lock her up". . . and put braces on her teeth. . . . We have a lot of fun with her.

"How do you suppose this change has come about," I mused. "I suppose part of it is the working towards having the baby—doing all that hard work. Or just the creating and seeing this thing come out of your own body in birth. And also partially because they are so helpless. There is no choice. I guess it is just that they are so helpless and you really feel that you have to care for them and also when she came out she was looking at both of us, very intelligently, almost as if she recognized us by our voices or something. It is just so overwhelming that you can't turn her down."

Susan

"It is worse than a headache. I must admit that it is worse than a headache." Susan is speaking about the pain. Before the birth she had wondered if the pain of childbirth could possibly be worse than the headaches she gets. Her headaches last for a day and a half sometimes and she manages so she hopes that labor will not be worse. But it is worse! "It is just more intense, quite a bit more. When they asked if I wanted something for the pain and Paul wondered if I wanted to wait, I just said, 'No, I don't want to wait.' So they gave me Demerol. But it doesn't take away the pain. It just made me woozy and sleepy in between."

Susan experienced the pain as low groin pain which radiated a little bit back into her hips, but not her back. And she didn't want anyone touching her. Although Paul was willing to rub her back or her shoulders, Susan could not stand it. So Paul helped her with her breathing. She said, "I'd look at him and he would help me out and do it, so it was really good—worked really well. And I kept trying to think about the baby coming out, that it [the cervix] is just opening up, that the pain is good. I kept trying to think it was positive."

Susan and Paul had waited so long for this baby. They had only been married three years but it seemed to Susan that having a child would just never happen. In fact, it was through having a uterine lining biopsy that Susan found out she was pregnant. She could not believe it! When they told her she was pregnant, Susan almost fell over! "I was in total shock because we had applied for adoption and were going to have the home visit in the summer. I had just finally decided that we wasted enough time waiting. It puts your whole life in a different perspective because you are constantly thinking, 'Maybe this month,' and you would get your hopes up, and I was tired of it. So the initial reaction was absolutely—I couldn't believe it!"

"Did you have any sensation that you were pregnant before this?" I wondered. "Well, the only thing I had noticed, and this had happened to me one other time, was that my breasts were really very, terribly sore. Like I couldn't run around, you know, couldn't go up and down the stairs. But this had happened once before and, oh no, I wasn't pregnant so when it happened this time, I was so fed up with my body not doing things right, that I thought, well, I'm not pregnant. I have a feeling, now, that I might have been pregnant before—but I don't know. I had said to Paul, 'I can't stand my body doing this, it does it all the time to me.' And he said, 'You think you are pregnant every two months, so don't worry about it, this always happens, and you are not, you know that'."

And then they found out she was!

Susan has striking coloring with fair skin and auburn hair. Just this year she had moved to teaching in a grade one class after many years of working with older children. She would never have made this move if she had known she would be pregnant as her work load doubled, especially during the first weeks of September. In the summer she had had the odd queasy day but generally felt good. "I have trouble with my legs, the joints, and in my back. I guess I notice that. And leg cramps, a charley-horse and it hurts the next day, it is so tender. But it is not bad. Maybe because we waited so long to get pregnant that I'd go through a lot before I would complain.

"It is really funny, I have always thought that pregnant ladies looked really great. It is not that I don't like how I look, but I am somewhat self-conscious at times. I wanted people to know that I was pregnant and not fat. And we went to a dance and I was wearing a sort of loose dress, and I felt funny dancing. I don't know why. It is not like I am humongous, you know, it was just sort of, I guess I felt a little self-conscious dancing."

The children in her grade one class were interested in her changing shape. Susan heard two little boys at the back of the room,

"I think she is having a baby."
"No, she is not. She is getting fatter."
"She isn't. She is not getting fat because getting fat is not a nice thing to say about ladies."

Susan was very conscientious about what she ate. "I really watch it. I feel guilty when I don't have my veggies for the day. But I also feel a little rebellious. There seems to be so much pressure from people that you have to do this, you have to do that—'How can you deprive your child?' I have quit drinking, and no coffee, and I had a can of Pepsi, and someone reminded me of the amount of caffeine in that, or I accidentally stood in front of the microwave, and it was 'Oh, my god, what are you doing standing in front of the microwave.' It is almost to the point where, 'For goodness sakes, guys, you know, one cup of coffee is not going to deform my child, or a half a beer.' It has gone to the extreme. But I am definitely trying to eat well. I've had lots of energy. It is much easier than I ever thought it would be. And I'm working harder than I've ever worked for a long, long time."

For Susan, too, clothes were troublesome. "Thank God I can sew my own clothes. My coloring makes it hard for me to wear reds and yellows and blacks—those are the big colors. This year royal blue is big, so everything is royal blue. In greens or beiges or browns or the colors I like, there is nothing. And a lot of them are 'cutsie', too. You know, things with buttons that say 'Baby.' And little frills and tucks and bows. You see, I think people notice you when you are pregnant, and I don't mind if I look okay but if I don't like what I am wearing, then I sort of feel self-conscious."

Early in her pregnancy Susan was concerned that she would not be able to stand up to her doctor, or that she would get worried if things were not happening when everyone said they should. She seemed to be more vulnerable than usual. "That is not how I was before, to get worried about every little thing. But now that I am pregnant, little things like that will get me wondering, 'Gee whiz, maybe they are right, maybe I should be feeling it move sooner.'

"And because I wanted to change doctors I was really wondering how I was going to tell this man." She wanted to change to a doctor who worked in a partnership so that she could be more sure of who would deliver her. She had heard that some of the doctors were "butcher types." A couple of her nurse friends had said, "Whatever you do, if your doctor is away, don't let these other guys deliver you. Oh, no, Susan, you can't, you can't let them deliver you!" They were worried about episiotomies ending up "at your kneecaps!" "Butcher types is how they were described," said Susan. "Well, I literally went into a panic. So I brought up my concern about who I would have if he wasn't there. And I was so pleased because the doctor just said, 'If it bothers you I could recommend you to a group of doctors and then you will know everyone.' He sort of gave me the go ahead, so I changed."

One Saturday, not long before Christmas, Susan again brought up this feeling of vulnerability. Paul was away for the weekend skiing. "This weekend it bothers me more than it normally would have. You see, he is gone and I can't get hold of him. I keep thinking, 'This is irrational, he's fine,' Yet I keep thinking, 'Oh dear, this baby needs a father—nothing better happen to him.' But he has always done this and it never bothered me before.

"And I panic a lot, I'm scared walking, slipping on the ice, and driving when it is really snowy. I've always been gutsy, it never bothered me. But now I think, 'Oh dear, what if I slipped off the road, or what if something happened.' I am just more conscious of it. At work they leave a space for me right in front of the door!" Susan had quit carrying out groceries. She had been getting spasms in her side that, at one point, kept her home for two days. She finally nailed down the cause. "I thought back to what I had lifted and realized I had carried some boxes with paper work and things. It wasn't like they were really heavy, but they were probably just straining me. So I quit going for groceries, and I really miss it!" she laughed.

It wasn't until Susan was into her eighth month of pregnancy that she let herself get excited about baby things. Earlier she had said, "It is just too early, like it is going to be jinxed. It is a silly feeling but"—however, now, that she had finished work she felt better about shopping for the baby. "And if worse came to worse and I delivered the baby now, there is a pretty good chance that, you know, things would be okay. Now I am going to sew curtains and make a comforter and that kind of thing."

When Susan talked about the pain, she really was concerned that she had not been too noisy and that she had been "good," that is, not "out of control." "I just didn't want to be yelling, and it was hard to judge how loud you are." Susan thought the birthing room was very cheerful, with its pretty wallpaper, rocking chair, coffee table, telephone, and new birthing bed. It was the first time the bed had been used, so the nurses, referring to the pamphlets, had Susan try different positions that could be accomplished with the various attachments on the bed.

"It was such a relief at that point to finally start pushing," Susan admitted. "They thought he'd be out a lot faster but the cervix was not retracting, so eventually the doctor decided to use forceps. So he gave me the needles and we got pushing again and I could feel where he was pulling—and there was suddenly a click, and he said, 'Well, you're doing it yourself now.' And the baby was born at a quarter after eleven and then I couldn't believe the sensation because—it was—as soon as I saw him, it was as if everything was gone. It gets very blurry. I guess it was unpleasant for a while. But it was a nice feeling that it was over. It was just mostly feeling him and seeing him. And the forceps marks are totally gone now. But I couldn't believe how blue he was. They tell you in prenatal classes how blue they come out, but he was BLUE . . . the little face was kind of purple and the rest was all blue. Paul was somewhat concerned about him, that he wasn't breathing okay, but they all said he was fine.

"I liked not having to be under blaring lights. When he was delivered, it was dark in the room except for a light for the doctor. It was a much softer experience than I expected. And they didn't rush the baby away but they brought him to me right away after they checked him out."

Again I wondered about the pain. "Does the pain of labor have any value?" "I think it was a useful experience," said Susan. "I would go through it again. I have no hesitation about that. And, at the time, I kept thinking that this is for the baby. I learned a lot more about Paul. We both said afterward that it was a love-deepening thing. That was one of the nicest things and a very good experience for both of us. I knew I loved Paul when I got married and I knew I loved him all the time, but I really knew why I loved him after we had this baby. So I think that is one of best things of the whole labor. And I learned about myself. I've gone through other painful situations. I was married before—and for a time I thought this was it—that I couldn't survive anymore. And now I look back at it and realize it was a positive growth situation for me. I look back on myself and can't believe how I used to be.

Anna

Anna and Bill had talked often about taking responsibility for the birth of their child. Their decision to have a home birth was carefully considered, weighing all the evidence for safety, as well as what seemed best to them. We had talked together in their home four or five times, and many times both Anna and Bill discussed their decision for home birth as a decision about responsibility. Bill said, "My sister, who was initially against the idea, is actually envious of us. She admires us for doing it, she thinks it takes courage. But we don't think it is taking courage, it is taking—what it really is—the ultimate in responsibility, that responsibility if something goes wrong. In a hospital there is always someone to attach responsibility or blame to. But if it happens at home, we will have to be responsible." Anna agreed, "I have thought of the potential of—let's say the baby doesn't make it—if it is in the hospital everyone would say that the doctor tried his very best, and if it should happen at home, we are going to be seen as irresponsible, and killers, and murderers. That is pretty drastic and I guess I am willing to live with that. I think we deny death. For how many people is death a real thing? How many have seen a dead person? Or touched a dead person? We have dehumanized death, just as hospitals have dehumanized birth through interventions, and goodness knows what else. I think that for us a birth at home is less of a risk than the hospital. People do not want to believe that it is safer at home because they want to put the responsibility into the hands of the doctor and the hospital. "Of course," she said later, "I would go to the hospital if I have to, but I really prefer not to."

So the talk was of responsibility and irresponsibility. Anna is used to taking responsibility for herself, "an adventurer" as she called herself. She described herself as being a rebellious teenager in a minister's family, being the only whites in a community in Western Samoa, taking a 5000-kilometer bicycle trip through Europe, and now, a home birth.

Bill and Anna are puzzled why so many people who talk in a negative way about their hospital experiences with childbirth still go back to the same situation the next time. Anna stated, "I think some of the negative experiences are because men are very protective or else they doubt our capabilities, and maybe that is why they are protective. I think it is all tied up in the man/woman relationship with man trying to be superior to woman and maybe envious of woman's capability to have children. Doctors/obstetricians often want to take credit for the delivery."

I asked Bill what he thought of Anna's suggestion that men really desire to be able to give birth. "Is that true for you? Do you feel that you would like to have the baby yourself?" Bill said he did not feel envious. He said, "I know that there is something going on there that I will never, never, know about. I think, sometimes I feel, that there is a bond being established right now that I, as much as I would like to, can't be a part of. Because it is just not possible." He looked to Anna. "But I like, by our closeness, to feel that I get a look, a see. There is always going to be something dear and special about a mother and child relationship, no matter what qualities I bring to it, it is something I can't hope to penetrate. I think that is the protectiveness that a lot of men have toward women." To this Anna reacted, "You see, I don't think that protectiveness is a valid, honest feeling for men to have, for the doctor to have, because, let's face it, women are built for the situation. The body takes care, the body does it all. We don't need episiotomies, we don't need enemas, we don't need to be shaved, the body takes care of it. And yet, man does all those things. The doctor is usually a man."

She continued, "I was thinking and talking to my mother about this. All the preparation for a home birth that we have to undergo is really good for us emotionally, psychologically, and even physically. We are responsible for getting the plastic sheet and sterilizing the towels. It has been good, even if to a certain extent you're overwhelmed with the responsibility. I guess I feel that I wouldn't encounter that responsibility if all you did was to pack your bag and go to the door of the hospital. It is a different kind of preparation.

"It is like immunization," said Anna. "Immunization is controversial. It is not as if we are not going to immunize, or want to be irresponsible. It is just that we are not going to accept something without question or research. We may come to the same conclusion, but at least it is our decision." She feels that generally one gets one's "knuckles rapped" for being skeptical.

She returned to the possibility of problems with the baby at birth. "One of the things you have to think about is if the child doesn't make it, is stillborn or . . . I think it would be better to be home, it is the best place to experience that, where you have your friends and your loved ones around with you. Birth and death are on a continuum, I think, and as hard as that would be, I'd prefer to be at home, and we have prepared for that.

"And then when she did come out, her face was quite blue. She was limp, had no reflexes, she didn't grimace or sneeze or do any of that kind of stuff. Her heart rate was good, but her respiration was irregular and slow and her color was blue. She didn't make any noise."

Anna was speaking about her newborn baby whom she held in her arms. Bill, Carol (her sister), Kate (Carol's eighteen-month-old daughter), and I were sitting in their home drinking coffee. Bill continued, "After she had the oxygen, she started breathing and sputtering and crying. Her Apgar score was only four at one minute. It was pretty scary. The midwife was very calm. She did what she had to do. But after it was all over, the midwife too was shaking."

Anna, in a calm voice, described what happened next, "Jena really recovered well, though. Within about two minutes she began to cry and that was just wonderful. We didn't even know whether she was a boy or girl at that point of time. She was on my tummy."

"It took a while to sort of get over that," said Bill. "I guess I thought that any breathing problems would be more a result of drugs in hospitals so I was really taken aback by all this. And I thought, 'Oh, my gosh, is this what having a kid is like? Terror like this? Will she be okay? Will she be okay tomorrow? Will she be okay the day after?' "

Katherine

We settled down in the living room, with a dish of cut up apples, nuts, and raisins. As I set up my tape recorder, I explained the nature of my study. Katherine was five months pregnant, wearing a maternity dress with tucks and ruffles at the neck. Her animated talk gave me the feeling that this pregnancy was good for her, and that she was enjoying herself. Her home, warm and inviting, displayed Indian hangings and oriental carpets giving a feeling of worldly experience. As we sipped raspberry tea she talked.

"I'm thirty-three now and up until I was twenty-five I would have said that I had too many other things to do, and then it seemed to me that the women that I knew who had children were in a disadvantaged position a lot of the time. As mothers, it seemed that all of a sudden their power or influence had really changed in society generally, as well as their relationships with their husbands."

Katherine had very deliberately chosen a line of work which she could rely on to support herself, and which would offer opportunities, as well as be adaptable to a woman's needs of child care responsibilities. When she had thought about what kind of studies to take, she looked for the kind of work that would offer the possibility of being in and out of the work setting. "I am not a career woman," she said emphatically, "in that I do not want to live the job, but I want to have a job that will fit into how I want to live." She goes on, "I was beginning to think of being a mother, but as well as being a mother, I wanted to maintain my independence both in this relationship and if this relationship didn't exist, I want still to be able to function on my own, and be able to bring up the kid."

She talked again about her friends who have children. "They were deeply involved in their children which really changed what they wanted to do and what they were able to do with their lives. I decided that for the next bit of time, say between twenty and twenty-five, I might be physiologically ready to have children, but mentally I was not. I had too many other things to do. I did a lot of traveling and had different jobs before I went back to school at twenty-six. And I wanted the job to fit into how I want to live, so I spent three years in pretty intensive schooling getting a degree which would, hopefully, make it easier for me to do what I wanted."

Katherine's man, Mike, had to be convinced that this was the time to have a baby. He had said to her at one point, "Well, you may be ready, but I am not absolutely ready at this time." So she described the waiting until he felt it was an okay time. She had said to him, "Look, I can't wait forever,

I don't mind waiting until you are ready, but please consider my situation. You can go on forever, but I can't! I thought that I should do something about it in the next couple years, or else it is going to get into a much more risky business, and I would prefer not to get into risk because ultimately the way I would like to go about having a baby is via a home birth, to make it as natural as possible." She backed this wish up by saying, "That is because I am not one that really enjoys a lot of interference in what I am doing in my life."

The decision to have a child was, as Katherine said, "a long time brewing." At one time she even thought that she might not want to have children. "But," talking so quietly that I could barely hear, "I just didn't want to say that, 'cause it doesn't even sound nice to say something like that. However it was something I thought about. I was making this decision about me, my body, and my life, and that was the way it was. But between twenty-five to twenty-seven, it was almost a biological thing, a real physical kind of feeling, and I know that sounds kind of hokey, but it was that my periods were something that were making me think, that each month my periods demonstrated that nothing had been done about that. Although I didn't want to do anything about it, I was thinking about it."

Eventually the time was right for her and Mike. "I had a really strong feeling before I missed my period. It was at that particular time in my cycle. It happened to be a particular cycle that we had had lots of good sex, and there was a change in my body, like I knew. I could feel the change in my breasts, a real change, and then I missed my period. That knowing made a difference. We had gone out for dinner and had wine with everybody else, and just because I had that feeling in me, that hunch, then obviously I couldn't, I shouldn't be drinking now. It would be an inappropriate thing to do." She kept the glass of wine in front of her because she did not want anyone to suspect her pregnancy, but she did not drink the wine.

Katherine was so sure of her pregnancy, that in buying the home pregnancy test, she opted for the "one-shot deal," rather than the one that contained two tests. Yet she wanted the doctor to verify it, too. She was nine weeks pregnant before her pregnancy was finally confirmed by the doctor. "It made it feel like, all of a sudden, the process was really under way, like things that I knew had to be sorted out, that had to be taken care of right away. At that visit, the doctor went over (with Mike and me), information about nutrition and supplements, about how to do perineal massage, and about breast preparation. I felt that he had looked me over, and that I was okay. I felt I was okay but it was good to hear it from someone else. Now, I knew it was real—like my body was telling me. But it is strange that you can't feel a thing. When you first feel movement that you know is decidedly nothing else but the baby, that is really, like you wait a long time for that confirmation that there is something that operates quite independently. It is just great.

"For a while it seemed that I only felt the baby when I laid down, when I was quiet. Now I can feel it anytime during the day, a lot of different times, but mostly when I lie down, and it is fun to watch my stomach change shape, and it is getting much more vigorous than it was. I haven't been able to isolate a heel or hand or head. I can't tell you where this kid is, I can't sort it out."

Katherine did not have the ultrasound test because there was no reason for it. While she thought it would be interesting, and did not think it would be harmful, she felt that since it had not been tested over a long period of time, and as it is not necessary, she would not have to have it done. She elaborated, "There are things that are meant to sort of be mysteries, that you don't know about, things that you can't be sure about." She was referring to the prebirth knowledge that some people have about the sex of the child. "It is interesting that I don't want to know. I don't feel that there is a need to know."

Later she said, "I am certainly aware of my pregnancy now. It is difficult not to think about it, because there is a lot of movement, you do have to go to the bathroom quite often, you are hungry, there are all sorts of little things that are saying that you are pregnant. A couple of times I haven't been able to get through a space even if I pull my stomach in. I am just too thick. I can't bend over easy—like putting on shoes. It is neat to have bigger boobs. I never knew what that was like—it is kind of funny! And the clothes. I began to realize that I had to get something. But I was shocked and dismayed. It is not like I am trying to hide my pregnancy but the clothes are huge, just bags—and they have little puffed sleeves. You really have trouble avoiding the bows, and the heavy duty gather, the sort of baby-fying clothes. I just don't want to look like that, to feel like that. In fact my boss, who is well aware that I am not very keen on having clothes that look 'the part,' said, 'Now don't you look sweet!' Teasing me because she knew I didn't like it."

Katherine talked about her decision to have a home birth. She said, "I really think of the home birth as a continuity in the way I live, that having my baby at home just makes sense. It seems to me that if you do believe birth is a natural process, then it can happen easier at home more naturally. It seems to make the whole thing more true." Her family questioned her about it. Her brother, a doctor, suggested to her that some people are electing cesareans when there is no "real" (that is, medical) reason. She said, "I thought that was illegal. The way he put it was that this child was a very special bundle, and this colleague didn't want to take any chances on a vaginal delivery and opted for a cesarean. He said there is not that much morbidity associated with a cesarean now. He made it sound like these colleagues of his perhaps valued their child more!" According to Katherine, "that is the ultimate in the medicalization, the technological kind of thing that really doesn't look at the whole picture—really a sad case."

In the talk about cesarean births, Katherine relayed the situation of a friend who had two children by cesarean section and was told that one does not really know what birth is like unless you have a vaginal birth. Katherine said, "I think that is a lot of hogwash because I know the relationship between you and your child starts with your pregnancy. A cesarean is kind of an interruption in that, but I am sure that you can establish as good if not better relationship with your child, mother/child kind of thing, afterwards. It doesn't depend, I don't think, on a vaginal birth."

Katherine's baby was born by cesarean after a labor of a couple of days. Her membranes had ruptured, yet her cervix had only dilated four centimeters. The surgery took place one stormy night a few days before Christmas. "And then when I was back in the room in the bed and people were attending me, cleaning up, taking blood pressure, and all this fuss and bother, Mike came in to see me and Mike told me that we'd had a girl and that she was eight pounds ten ounces and I remembered that I had been told, but it hadn't registered. Mike said, 'You can see the baby if you want,' and I said, 'I can't.' I just didn't have the energy." At that point it was hard enough to focus on Mike and respond to him. "He was leaning over the bed and beaming and said that she was lovely and that everything was fine and she was under a lamp to keep warm."

Katherine did not see Brett until the next morning. "When I first saw her, and the nursery nurse was a little bit concerned about leaving this baby with me because I was a cesarean she double-checked and double-checked the tags. . . . I was waiting for this lady to go away so I could grab this baby and have a look at her.

Later she said, "When I first saw her I was really surprised at what she looked like—I didn't know what to expect—I guess I expected a fair child, she is dark; and I didn't expect such a big baby. Her face and her big chubby cheeks were really a surprise. I think that probably the real feeling [of mothering] happened over that first day. At first I think I was just too curious. I just looked at her as an object to examine and see all that is there, but then after a while, just being able to comfort her. That is, if I talked to her she seemed to be soothed. She seemed to know somebody was there. When you get a response from the child to something that you're doing, that feels motherly then. Maybe that is when you start feeling it.

"I pricked Brett with a pin a couple of days ago," confessed Katherine when the baby was about two months old. "It was terrible. I was morose the whole afternoon. I felt so bad!" It took Brett a while to react and for Katherine to realize what had happened. "She went to sleep when she finally did settle down exhausted from crying, and I couldn't wait for her to wake up again so I could hold her and say, 'It's okay, I'm sorry.' "

We talked about the cesarean. "When I think about the cesarean I wonder 'Why?'—why it went that way—what was I doing or what was I not doing? Again it is kind of a guilt thing. As I say, I've apologized to her I don't know how many times—'I'm sorry kid, that it happened like that.' I am trying to find out more about it from John [the doctor]. I want to know what the obstetrician wrote. I want to know why it was necessary to do it. I want to know her Apgar score. Perhaps there is a little bit of sadness that it happened that way, and there is a real sense, when you have a cesarean, of the inadequacy of your body. It didn't work right!"

Then Katherine told of the sense of uncomfortableness around people who knew she had planned things differently. She said, "One of the girls said to me, 'Could I be frank with you? I don't know what to say to somebody when they've had a cesarean birth. Do you say too bad or congratulations or what?' And I said, 'You can say congratulations about the baby, but it is too bad that you had to have a cesarean.' As far as I am concerned, it is too bad, but that is the way it went and it is too bad."

I wondered how things have changed for Katherine. She said, "I've got Brett on my mind all the time—whatever I am planning to do. It's on-going. It's fragmented my thinking. For example, if I am watching the news and she is awake, I can't pay really good attention—or when I am on the phone. If she needs me for whatever reason, or if I am aware of her, other things have to go. I guess I think that mothers live a very fragmented existence."

She talks of going back to work in the Fall. In addition to thinking about the child care arrangements and how she will work and still spend enough time with her baby, she also wonders how having a baby will affect her work. "Although I am not very career minded, I find that when I have a special project going I become quite involved with it. I don't know whether or not some of the ways I've responded to things at work might change because I have a baby at home who has more priority than the job." Yet she wondered, "You never get paid in money—that is with any official recognition—for what you do as a mother. And you do a lot. I don't want to think of it like 'work' because it is all tied up in loving your baby, loving and caring for your baby. Perhaps there has got to be enough intrinsic reinforcement of what you are doing or things may just get out of focus. I can't feel too strongly about that right now, but I sure can see how it might happen, that you start feeling, 'Why did I buy into this one?' "

THE TEXTURE OF CHANGE

Women move to motherhood in a linear way, through the nine-month pregnancy, the twelve-hour labor, the forty-five second contraction, the slow, painful, passage of the baby through the birth canal, the timeless wait for the first breath, the momentous reaching to take the baby, and the twenty-hour day, seven-day week of life with the child. But on another level, this movement is not linear. A linear view does not account for the intertwining of the growing, accommodating, and birthing woman's body and her developing relationship with the child she carries within and to whom she extends her arms at birth. A linear view does not accommodate the depth of change that such a transformative process entails. New experiences reach back to earlier experiences which are now understood in a different modality. Similarly, experiences earlier in the pregnancy reach forward to envelop present experiences with transformed significance. Thus transformation takes linear time but involves change that is deep, complex, and dramatic. The move from woman to mother can be profound, and may, as Neumann (1955: 32) suggests, "reshape the woman's life down to its very depths." "Having a child drastically changes the lives of most women, opening up previously unimagined new selves, new areas of responsibility, delight, exhaustion, anxiety, ambivalence, and physiological change" (Morgan 1984: 223).

Women expect to be different as mothers. In fact, they are continually reminded by everyone that their lives will never be the same again: They will never have a night's sleep, never be able to go to movies, never be free to live their own lives. In pregnancy women worry about this change. They wonder about their changing relationships with the men and women in their lives—their friends—their own mothers. They begin to feel their dependence and vulnerability. They wonder about their ability and their energy. They fear that their bodies will age and sag. They wonder if they will be ready when their "time" comes. They even wonder if they will love their child. Yet, as they express these fears they also hope for change, as Jane said, "I never really liked children, but everyone assures me that you will like your own" (J1). They hope they will be transformed so they can be the mothers they want to be.

Brenda's experience of her impending motherhood places the concept of transformation, itself, into questioning relief. *What is meant by transformation?* How did Brenda enter a transformative experience? Was she open to the experience so that her life was changed? Brenda was inhabited by a child before she seemed ready. When her baby girl was born she could not immediately reach out to her. Earlier in pregnancy she said that she should be exactly as she was before, "I want my own life too, like if I want to go out for an evening with my friends, I should be able to" (B1). Even before pregnancy she and her husband decided that they should not change their whole life because of a child. "We should change some things, yes, but you have to be yourself or you would be at each other's throat. It would be more of a chore than a blessing" (B1). Brenda had wanted a boy. It took her some time to accept her baby girl. Almost a week after the birth she admitted to still calling her baby "Kevin," and referring to "her" as "him" (B3). She said that Tom, her husband, tells her she is a terrible mother. "But, it just doesn't want to go through my head that she's ours and she's a girl and not a 'Kevin.' "Then she looked at her baby and said, "But we'll keep you, right?" Two months later Brenda still is aware that the change that is expected of her is slow in coming. She said, "I don't talk about Suzie unless I'm asked. A lot of people are upset because I don't carry a picture of her around. And a lot of people get upset because I call her a 'kid.' But I'm not going to change overnight" (B4). But then, eight months later, she can say to her pregnant friends who worry about becoming mothers, "You change, just give it time, it will come. Before it was, 'I want to be a mother but I want to be myself.' Now I figure that I am myself and I am a mommy" (B5). And she is pregnant again, excited about the next child, feels well, and even looks forward to the birth (B6).

It seems possible that the transformation from woman to mother is suspended for some women, taking longer for them than for others, varying in intensity and depth. For Brenda, although she could not deny the reality of pregnancy, said, "I don't want to be a mom just like that" (B1). Neither could she deny the reality of the child born to her, yet she said "no" at the time of birth (B3). How many women say "no" at different points in their own experience, and feel ambivalent about the magnitude of change in their lives? Is it possible that all women sometimes say no? Or is it possible that some women always say "no"? Is it possible that they cling to their familiar life because of fear, refuse to take on the necessary challenges that come with having children? Are there some women who are unable to receive new life, either for the child or for themselves?

Phyllis Chesler in her book *With Child* wrote to her child:

> Last year I died. My life without you ended. Our life together—only nine months!—ended too: abruptly and forever, when you gave birth to me. Being born into motherhood is the sharpest pain I've ever known. I'm a newborn mother, your age exactly, one year old today. (1979: 281)

Chesler's language of transformation is dramatic. The woman died when the mother was born. The pregnant woman was transformed too: the symbiotic togetherness ended. The separation was painful—a sharp pain. An Abyssinian woman reminds us of the extent of the impact this transformation has for women:

> The woman conceives. As a mother she is another person than the woman without child . . . . Something grows into her life that never departs from it. She is a mother. She is and remains a mother even though her child dies, though all her children die. For she at one time carried the child under her heart. (Meltzer 1981: 3)

To become a mother is a change which may be more complex and overwhelming than any other social transition. It changes one's life forever.

> Through you, Ariel, I'm enlarged, connected to something larger than myself. Like falling in love, like ideological conversion, the connection makes me *feel* my existence. (Chesler 1979: 246)

There are mysteries surrounding the transformation of woman to mother which cannot, and, perhaps should not, be articulated. It is necessary, rather, to treasure the mystery while we try to grasp what can be revealed. Becoming a mother involves a movement from one mode of living to another; from woman without child to woman with child. That is straightforward, no mystery there. But attention to the "movement" itself, the movement from one form of life to another, may reveal elements of transformation which are contained within the mystery—or perhaps it is a magic that is tied to the wonder at the strength of our relationship to our children.

> Woman necessarily experienced herself as subject and object of mysterious processes and as a vessel of transformation. The mysterious occurrences in her body, the instinctual mysteries of her existence, are exclusively the possession of woman. (Neumann 1955: 291)

The changes that occur in a woman as she births a child—that connection to a reality larger than herself—is a connection that is felt through living as mother. On the one hand, in recognizing the mystery and awe of giving birth and becoming a mother, there is the inherent danger of seeing the activity of reproduction as the "major identifying characteristic of female human beings, and indeed our primary reason for existing," which Morgan (1984: 41) argued can lead to disregarding women's "authentic human rights and powers." On the other hand, acknowledging and accepting the mystery can remind women of the magnitude and sacredness that being a mother entails—as bringers of life to children and to society.

The experience of childbirth ties women to the fundamental cycle of life: birth, death, and re-birth. I remember very poignantly the death of my father at the time when my daughter was three months old. Her coming (her presence) helped to bear the pain of his going (his absence). My being a mother assured that life would go on. "The old cycle repeats itself again and again. . . . Nature goes on repeating itself but there is no end to its infinite variety and every spring is a resurrection, every new birth a new beginning . . . it becomes a revival of ourselves and our old hopes centre round it . . ." (Sorel 1984: 27).[1] But "becoming a mother," is more than a revival of ourselves, that is, a living on through our children. Becoming a mother shows, perhaps, the possibility of renewed life through birth, not only of our children but of ourselves. Is it possible that as a woman becomes a mother she can truly become herself?

This book explores woman's transformation to mother during a short period in a woman's life—over the period of pregnancy and the first few months of caring for the child. This does not mean that the process of transformation is a succinct experience. Rather transformation may be a never ending process, changing and developing each moment in the lives of women with children of varying ages—in the womb, infant, school age, adolescent, or adult. "In a very immediate and day to day way women live change," said Miller (1976: 54). They change with their growing and developing children. Gaining a better understanding of this dynamic process which occurs in women who mother can give clues to understanding a learning experience appropriate for all people living in a rapidly changing atmosphere of the present age. Such a learning process might uphold "growing" as opposed to "aging"—if we just learn how (Ruddick 1983: 219). Yet the intense period of pregnancy and birth is a time of deep change, as Chesler (1979: 164) so vividly exclaimed, "Women, Do you think I'm not drowning in this transformation to mother?" Or as another mother said, "My daughter has changed part of my understanding so radically that I have difficulty recognizing who I was before" (Dowrick and Grundberg 1980: 79). Susan, too, said, "I look back on myself and can't recognize how I used to be" (S4).

WEAVING THE FABRIC

Wherein does this transformation reside? Where does transformation begin? Is there a beginning? One way of conceptualizing the beginning of transformation is to examine the experiences and relations that are involved in the decision to have a child. With Christine we are confronted by the decision or the resolve to have a baby. *What is the nature of the experience of decision?* Is the resolve (and the planning that ensues from it) already a significant element of the transformation? How was Christine's resolve a real commitment? Christine said "yes" to a child in her life but when the child did come—and there was the possibility of miscarriage—Christine's managerial decision to have a child was questioned in a different light. How is the decision to have a child already a transforming experience?

For Jane, the focus seemed to be on the "presence" of the child in her body. *How is the presence of the child experienced?* Through seeing and knowing the child and her changing body, Jane began to see and know herself as a mother. Through the interrelatedness with the child in pregnancy, at birth, and in daily care, a woman begins to see herself as mother. How does the interaction with the child transform a woman to motherhood?

Birth is a separation of mother and baby. Susan's story is suggestive of the paradox of separation that brings integration and wholeness into her life. *What is the nature of separation that leads to integration?* What part does a woman's reproductive labor play in this move to wholeness? What is the role of pain in this transformation? How is birthing pain experienced?

Next comes Anna's story. Anna showed that the decision to experience pregnancy and birth entails responsibility. How is responsibility experienced? To decide to be responsive in a deep sense to life with children is to be open to its terror and possibilities. But does Anna realize this aspect of responsibility until she is transformed through life experience? *What is the nature of taking on the responsibility of motherhood?* What is it like to take responsibility that terrorizes one? What is it like to be responsible for that which is beyond control?

Katherine's story reveals that transformation to motherhood involves a self-questioning and a disruption of previously held self-assuredness. She talks of self-guilt, of wondering how she will be competent now that this child is on her mind. She is even rushed home by thoughts of her child. *What is the experience of having a child on one's mind?* Is there the possibility of the losing of self in the move to motherhood? How can one lose oneself to another, and yet be oneself?

These moments will be used to bring to light aspects of the transformative experience of childbirth. The complex pattern of movement from woman to mother shows itself in the development of each moment. In a sense, each individual thematic moment reveals the transformative process. Without fragmenting the process into different stages, each moment is an example of one way to look at the process. At the same time, however, all the moments together uncover more clearly the whole picture. I think of a small crystal which sits on my desk. As I look through the crystal head-on there are dark spots through which I cannot see. In order to see more clearly the crystal must be turned a bit to allow me to see well from that one angle. Again, I must turn the crystal to bring to light another point of view. So it is with the identified moments of the transformative experience of motherhood. While overlapping, each moment reveals the process from a slightly different perspective, bringing aspects into focus which could not be previously seen. Yet, at the same time, each moment casts its shadow and its reflection on the other moments.

The existential themes of time, space, body, and relationship provide a structure into which the story moments are woven in order to describe the reality women experience with the birth of their first child. The attempt is to weave the threads of these themes and moments into an experiential fabric which describes the transformative process. Such a weaving creates a text that will have its own design, dependent on the colors and textures of the threads, and the inspiration and skill of the weaver. Although the pattern is individual, in a sense a creative work, the whole may bring a clearer understanding of the meaning of being a mother. The phenomenological approach used here is not immune to critique. It simply is the best way I know at present to construct a narrative that through its mimetic textual quality allows us to return to experience in an enriched fashion. The next five chapters take a closer look at these thematic moments as women move to motherhood.

Chapter 3

The Beginning: The Transformative Experience of the Decision to Have a Child

THE MEANING OF DECISION

"The deep personal significance of the decision of whether or not to have children [is] the most irrevocable and important one that most of us will make" (Dowrick and Grundberg 1980: 8). Christine (and her husband) thoughtfully made the decision to have a child. But as she reflected on her resolution Christine also sensed her own indeterminacy about the meaning of the decision. She said:

> You think about it. You *think* you want to be a parent. You *think* that it will be a neat thing. You *think* it will give you the positive feedback that a career can give. But you don't know. You have to find out. (C7)

A woman decides on motherhood. What does it mean to understand such a decision as decision?

In a pamphlet "Having a Child . . . Is it for Us?" made available by the Planned Parenthood Association, the seriousness of the decision to have a child is emphasized. Such a decision "deserves to be arrived at only after a careful look at the adjustments that must be made." One is encouraged to ask oneself questions like: "Does having and raising a child fit in the life I want to live?" "What can I get out of it?" "What is there to know about kids?" These questions relate to one's job, goals, energy, leisure-time, finances, and priorities. One is encouraged to explore one's reasons for wanting a child: "To give someone the opportunities I never had?" "To have a child to be like me?" "To keep me company?" "To pass on beliefs, values, and ideas to?" "To prove my femininity?" One is encouraged to ask oneself: "Do I enjoy being with kids?" "Do I like teaching?" "How do I handle angry feelings?" or "How do I feel about getting up at night?"

The problem of decision making about motherhood is very real for women in present day society (Fabe and Wikler 1979). In the past, there may not have been a "real" decision, maybe one just accepted (or rejected) what nature (God) brought. Of course, women in earlier times did make decisions about children, as evidenced by the number of "back-room" abortions, or the fluctuations of birth rates during differing economic and social circumstances. Modern contraception forces women, as never before, to respond to the question of children in their lives. Some women try to ignore it; some put it off until it is too late; and others panic and end up with the "symbolic child" (the child that is conceived because of fear that life is passing by rather than because of a desire for a child)(Fabe and Wikler 1979). Some live to regret what might have been—to regret the personal disappointment of being childless (Greer 1984).

Fabe and Wikler (1979: 263) said that the most important question to be dealt with in the decision of whether or not to have a child is "How much do I really want a child?" This question should be confronted head-on. Psychotherapy, couple therapy, getting more exposure to children, and insights gleaned from imagining life with children, are tools suggested to assist in facing this question. But how can one know what it means to have a child before one has a child? How can one even know what it means to want a child?

The question of wanting a child reveals a significant dilemma. Many women who have children speak of their own personal, profound, and inmost change. They discover commitments of which they did not know themselves capable. They find a happiness they never dreamed possible—like the woman who thought being a mother would be stultifying yet found it "exotic." The childless woman is totally ignorant of this knowledge. She cannot know. To ask: "How much do I really want a child?" is to really ask, "How much do I desire a new responsibility which may commit me in a way I cannot now possibly fathom?"

I think there is something called the nesting syndrome. It just hits people. Many who said they would never settle down, never have kids, all of a sudden at twenty-nine or thirty seem to want to settle. (J1)

It was always a consideration, just a matter of when. A lot of things came into the consideration—finances, job security, the fact that we love to travel, the question of bringing a child into *this* world—being torn between those things and thinking that we would be good parents and me desperately wanting to be a mother. I know it is right. I think there is a yearning for a woman to be a mother. (A1)

It was always sooner or later. We have been married five years, we have our house, have our dogs, have our vehicles, it is more or less time. (B1)

Really it is a biological thing, a real kind of physical feeling. My periods were something that were making me think—each month my periods demonstrated that nothing had been done about that . . . . It was something that suddenly became a strong basic urge. (K1)

We talked about it. Yes, we wanted to have children. However, then when we decided to have a child, it was a different story. Then we had problems getting pregnant. (S1)

There are inner considerations, such as the yearning for a child, the desire to settle, or the nesting syndrome; there are outer considerations of "having a house," of finding the right time, and the reality of getting pregnant. Do these notions speak to the question of "How much do I want a child?" To yearn implies a sense of longing for something, a need for fulfillment perhaps. Does having a child fulfill? Does a child help one settle? Does "having a house" allow one to think about children? What if the child does not come? Will one then want a child more? And what about the child who comes when the woman does not want a child at all?

Think back to Christine's story. Christine handled her decision making very deliberately. She wanted a child enough to stop using contraception. She wanted a child enough to hire a mediator to reduce the tension between her and her husband in making the decision. She became pregnant just as she had planned. It was a rational process. Or was it? She started to bleed. There was a chance she would lose the child. She had experienced, in some way, the presence of the child—so that the thought of not having a child took on a different meaning for her. It almost seemed as if the child was deliberating about her as well. Having experienced the child's presence, Christine could now experience the absence. She could no longer think of her life without a child. She had chosen. The very circumstance of the choosing the child had changed her life forever. All her previous rational deliberations lost their relevance—she is caught by life, so to speak. She was captured by the very presence of the child.

Let us listen to two other voices. Judy Chicago, a woman who is dedicated to articulating the experience of women in birth through her art, does not have a child. She said, "I have almost never really allowed myself to need another person, to depend upon another person. I've always deprived myself of that so as not to get 'caught.' But I understand how one can be caught by life. It is something most women seem to both crave and fear" (1985: 34). Oriana Fallaci, who became pregnant by mistake, said:

> I am locked in fear. I am lost in it. It is not fear of others. I don't care about others. It is not fear of God. I do not believe in God. It is not fear of pain. I have no fear of pain. It is fear of you, of the circumstance that wrenched you out of nothingness to attach yourself to my body. (1976: 9)

Both women want to "make it alone." They do not need others. They do not need the "Other," in this case, the child. Does Chicago truly realize the deep truth of her deprivation—of not allowing herself to need another? Does Fallaci really stand so alone in the world? By the very fact of pregnancy, in the fear of the child, does not Fallaci display her deep fear of (and therefore belief in) the Other, pain, and God? Chicago and Fallaci, in "making" a decision against children do so with a sense of clarity that is eroded with the subtle notion that such clarity may also be a false clarity. Something else is at stake—the circumstance that attached the baby to one's body—the sacredness—the being "caught by life."

The voices of Fallaci and Chicago, as well as the other voices that talk of the house, the right time, or even the settling and yearning, are not animated by the deep knowledge of what it is like to have children in one's life. But they are suggestive of the possibility of something beyond the rational "making up of one's mind." The voices suggest the possibility of change in one's life that could be good, overwhelming, and, yes, fearful. There is a "searching for life" in the quality of the talk.

The Latin origin of the word "to decide" comes from *dēcīdere* meaning "to cut off," which contains the sense of cutting off possibilities with decision making. On the one hand, we see the decision to have a child as one that will cut off possibilities in life—of "being gobbled up," being "bogged down," "losing oneself," "putting one's relationships in jeopardy," or "being dependent." On the other hand with the choice for the child, there is something else at stake, the possibilities—the opening up, being enriched, being blessed.

"Are you sorry you did it?" she asks. Intelligently. Urgently.

"Yes," I answer. "I'm trapped." I can't take Ariel back, or move away from him.

A long silence.

"No," I say, "I'm blessed now."

(Chesler 1979: 182)

When mothers speak about motherhood they may sound ambivalent. Perhaps this is due to the paradox which takes decision making about children beyond the rational. It is being caught by life. "No wonder women don't hear what mothers say until afterward, when they hear themselves speaking as mothers" (Chesler 1979: 182). So instead of the deliberate, rational "making" of decision, "the thinking about it," which sounds like a technical process or instrumental reasoning (supported by the mechanism of decision making—a cost-benefit analysis), there is a notion of "coming to" decision. Such a notion is, in a sense, like Kierkegaard's "leap of faith"—a realization that having a child opens one to life's possibilities—which can only be taken with "fear and trembling" (Olson 1986). Such a decision cannot be fully understood until the child is concretely, by choice, in one's life.

THE TIME OF DECISION

It seemed that Christine and her husband came to the decision when the counselor mediated their tension enough for "the situation to resolve itself." Yet later, Christine recognized that she had, in her heart, already opened herself to the thought of a child in her life but decided that if her husband did not agree she would continue to say "no." Although she wanted to have a career and had spent many years developing that, the possibility of children was always there. So it may be that the choice to have a the child was already made—the deliberation, the decision making came later. It appeared to be different for Nathan. For him a child could wreck everything—the good life that he and Christine had. Christine thought it was the difference in their family backgrounds. She describes what she said was an excellent childhood:

> I saw in my parents that having children had been a good thing in their lives—had really fulfilled them. I had happy relationships all through my childhood, so I didn't see having children as a negative thing—just a matter of the right time. (C1)

So for Christine, the decision was not whether or not she wanted children, but was, rather, whether or not the two of them wanted children. In fact, she said later, that if they had decided against children, she would have grieved for the children she would not have. She was open to children in a way that Nathan was not.

Jane and Brenda, on the other hand, were not as open to children as their husbands were. For Brenda it was much too soon, a shock: "Here I am going to be a mom and I don't want to be a mom just like that. Thank God, it takes five or six months before you really start to show" (B1). Until the baby starts to show itself to others, a woman can deny it to herself. Having already said "yes" to a child, there are still times when the very decision may be questioned. Jane, already six months pregnant, experiences times when she doubts about whether she wants to be a mother: "I'm not sure I want to give up my freedom . . . and I don't really like kids" (J1). Recall Jane's description of the incident at the restaurant where she worked. She said, "I took the baby, which I would never do in my life, because I don't like kids and I don't like dirty kids" (J1). Moved by that experience in a way that surprised her, Jane, through her own pregnancy, felt herself opening her life to other people's children and to the possibility of a child of her own.

It may not be possible to pinpoint the moment of decision, if indeed there is such a moment. The decision may come when a woman is "up against the clock" like Christine, who says she does not want to reach thirty-six or thirty-seven and find out the decision has already been made (Fabe and Wikler 1979; Russell and Fitzgibbons 1982). For another, the decision may begin in the back of her mind as a girl playing dolls with her friends, as a young woman menstruating for the first time, or as an adult imagining a child at her breast or reaching to take a sweet-smelling baby from a friend. Yet, for another, like Katherine, it may not truly come until she takes her own baby into her arms and begins care on a daily basis, "when the baby seemed to be soothed by the sound of her voice" (K3). And still, the decision may not be fully realized until the child is sick and the woman is overwhelmed with a sense of what it would mean to lose this child. Then again, it may begin at all these times, experienced by feeling the urge to hold, to stroke, and to nurture the child, with increasing depth and commitment at various times in a woman's life. Of course, there is the possibility that a decision may never be fully accepted at all.

EMBODIED DECISION

Time is running on—relentlessly. Thirty seems to be the magic number these days. That is, if women have not had a child before thirty some feel that time is beginning to run out. "Once I came to thirty, there was a sense of urgency," said Christine (C1). "I am thirty-three and my biological clock is running out. It starts becoming a risky business," felt Katherine (K1). "We are getting older, I'm thirty-one and Paul is thirty-four," Susan (S1) acknowledged. "While I don't want to be too young either, you know, the maturity factor, but," said Anna (A1), "I still don't want to be a grandparent either." Even Brenda, at twenty-six, felt that if she was going to have two children, she should do so before she reached thirty. She said this in spite of her awareness that the available technology reduces the problems associated with later first-time pregnancies (Fabe and Wikler 1979: 279–88). The other women, aged between twenty-nine and thirty-three, agreed.

It was Katherine (K1) who said that each month her menstrual period demonstrated to her that nothing had been done about her decision to have a baby. The monthly rhythm of her female body, her woman's body, her bleeding, reminded her that time was passing. Susan (S1) was constantly thinking, "Maybe this month!" The rhythm of women's bodies forces them to wonder about the time for having children. They are forced to attend to the question of the "right" time. In the recognition that the decision to have a child is, for women, a bodily one, Katherine's reaction to her own menstrual bleeding becomes more understandable.

Menstrual blood is the sign of hope and the promise of children. Neumann in discussing the archetypal[1] nature of the feminine, refers to the mysteries of transformation as primarily blood-transformation mysteries which lead women to experience their own creativity. Menstruation is the first blood-transformation mystery in women—in every respect more significant than the first emission of sperm by the man—and rightly regarded as an important moment in the life of the female (Neumann 1955: 31). The blood of menstruation is truly the blood of life. One wonders why it is so often thought of as "the curse." Perhaps it is because aspects of body, especially the bodily experiences of women, are often regarded as taboo in this society. Think of how information about menstruation is predominantly seen in terms of protection, cleanliness, and effort to carry on with "normal" activities. In fact, the underlying effort is that no one will suspect that a woman is menstruating. Yet, menstruation, while reminding Katherine that nothing has be done about her decision to have a child, is also the outward sign of the potential for children and the continuance of life.

THE SPACE OF DECISION

World as Home for a Child

Does one want to continue this world? The question of bringing a child into *this* world was a factor to be considered in the decision for both Anna and Jane. This world of nuclear shadows, of poverty, of sadness, causes women to feel fear. Yet for the women and men who decide to become parents, it seems that the world, as a space for children, is seen differently than before. "There was a general feeling among people that I grew up with," said Jim, Jane's husband, "that it wasn't a very good world into which to bring a child. But you change, just all of a sudden, and I don't remember it actually happening, the flipping . . . it is more of an understanding of what it is all about" (J1). Is this what Jane called the nesting syndrome? What makes people want to "settle"?

In exploring this attitudinal flip/flop, this changed attitude toward the world that makes it possible to choose to have a child, I was attracted by Bachelard's image of nests. He said:

A nest . . . is a precarious thing, and yet it sets us to *daydreaming of security*. . . . And so when we examine a nest, we place ourselves at the origin of confidence in the world, we receive a beginning confidence, an urge toward cosmic confidence. Would a bird build its nest if it did not have its instinct for confidence in the world? . . . The nest . . . know[s] confidence in the world . . . The nest . . . knows nothing of the hostility of the world. (1969: 102–3)

The image of the world as a "nest" calms our fears. In the act of conceiving a child (into the "nest" of the womb) we show confidence in the world as a good place to be, and we are tuned to it in a new way. The changed attitude may, thus, come first. We see the world as a world for children and are prepared to conceive a child. Or it may be the converse: In deciding on children we come to accept the world as a place for children, and begin to take responsibility for the world in a different way.

Chesler (1979) said that when we choose the existence of a child, in spite of what we know about the world, we accept our own existence. Through acceptance of our own existence, which comes with maturity, we come to realize "what it is all about." According to Arendt (1961), this acceptance of responsibility for the world and for ourselves is the essential condition needed for people to become parents, the right to "summon" children into life through conception and birth. In accepting a child in our life, we are compelled to face our world in a new way, and to take responsibility for it. Jane's husband, telling of his changing view of the world, described the following scenario. "A woman comes up to the bar, obviously pregnant, and orders a zombie, or something else with a lot of liquor in it. What does a bartender do" (J1)? It became a moral issue for Jane's husband, an issue that has him taking responsibility for the world in a way that he did not before he decided to bring his own child into the world.

House as Home for a Child

It was in the women's homes where we talked about becoming mothers. With Christine, we met in her office on two occasions, but it was *her* office, with the door closed and with the request to "hold" calls. It was not a public place. Does it suit the nature of the talk that it should be done at home? Could it not have been done in a restaurant? Or a mall? Yet, the private space of home seems the best place to talk about "motherhood." It is to this house that we bring the child. What is so necessary about a house as a place to talk of childbearing and mothering? What is so important about the house?

Brenda said, "We have our house, our vehicles, our dogs, so it is more or less time" (B1). On first thought, this may seem like a materialistic and inappropriate approach in the consideration of bringing a child into one's life. But what is really being said? What does having a house have to do with having a child? Bachelard likened the house to a cradle. "Life begins well, it begins enclosed, protected, all warm in the bosom of a house" (1969: 7). The house has the power to integrate thoughts, memories, and one's dreams. The house is the environment where we participate in the original warmth, a "well-tempered matter of the material paradise." The house holds childhood, maternally "in its arms." Having "our house" gives security to women, a place of protection and confidence. It is now the right time to think of a child. But what does it mean to have a house? And what does having a house have to do with making a decision about children?

We have all experienced coming home after a day's work in the outside world—or shopping—or traveling. Have we not often heard, "The best thing about going away is coming home?" I remember, as a child, how my brothers and I, as we neared our hometown, would crane our necks to be first to yell out, "I see the water-tower!" And remember the feeling of seeing "our" house as we turn the corner of our street? "Home" takes on a special loveliness when one returns after a long absence. It always looks more beautiful than I expect, the hardwood floors covered with the rugs made by my husband's grandmother, the oak table, the tea cozy that brings warm thoughts of shared times with friends, our bed that allows sleep to come more easily. Even the carelessly thrown books and boots of the children are less troublesome than usual. I am "at home" here. This place is my shelter, my dwelling place. Here, I can be myself. When we have a home, we can think of having a child.

Carrying a child, Anna searched for a new place to live. For her, an apartment was no longer appropriate, for she was planning a home birth. "Simply because of the neighbors," she said, "It would be an intrusion to them, our sounds imposed on them, whether the baby's cry, or, God knows, I'm a screamer, and who knows what is going to happen when I give birth" (A1). But maybe there is more to it than noise. Images of houses are stabilizing and by living in such images, there is space to think about a new life, a life that would be our own, that would belong to us in our very depths. It may also have to do with the need for privacy during intimate and personal events. It may be that the idea of having a home for a child is an attitude, a commitment to be "at home" for a child.

SHARING THE DECISION

A decision without action is not truly a decision. With the decision to have a child, action involves the discontinuance of birth control methods—stopping the pill, removing of the IUD, "forgetting" to put in the diaphragm. For some, like Christine, it meant charting her temperature to identify the day of ovulation, and the most promising time of conception. In all situations, deciding on a child includes heterosexual intercourse (or artificial insemination)—a relational activity.

Good Sex

What does "good sex," that Katherine talked about, have to do with coming to decision? Is there something special about the love making when it contains the possibility of making a child? We know that sexuality encompasses the processes of childbearing, birth, and commitment to the baby and need not be reduced just to coitus, but that may be easy to forget. With the pleasures of sexual intercourse without the fear or possibility of pregnancy (due to the increasing use of birth control methods), the procreative potentiality of "good sex" may be forgotten. Yet many women remember the moment of conception. The sexual act can overwhelm us, putting us in touch with a larger nature sensed by the merger and disruption of our discrete existence (Kittay 1983). Childbirth is still more powerful, at least for women who are willing, awake, and not terrorized by fear. "The uterine contractions that are needed to expel the baby are far more intense than orgasmic contractions; and the tiny head emerging from within us remains a magical conjuring act which discloses our continuity amid discreteness as completely as any sexual encounter" (Kittay 1983: 118). "Good sex" or "having a go" as Anna put it, with the purpose of willing procreation, ties women's sexual nature very concretely to childbearing. The possibility of childbirth, itself, as a sexual experience, an orgasmic experience, is a real one. Of course, conception can also be a "mistake." But many women, even then, remember the time. Perhaps it was an especially passionate encounter—as when a couple is together after a long absence—when birth control methods are forgotten or neglected. It may be completely "wrong" at first, so the decision to have the child is made following conception rather than before. For the woman, already on the road to motherhood, it may be extremely difficult. This happened to Paula—and now that Joanna is over four years old Paula cannot imagine what life would be like without her (P3).

We begin to see the problem of trying to separate into discrete themes a process that can not be broken down into fragments. A discussion of "good sex" is as much a part of the decision to have a child as it is to the whole experience of pregnancy, and the birth, itself. Good sex, conception, pregnancy, and childbirth are all part of a woman's sexual nature, and are integral to the transformative process. Becoming a mother is therefore a sexual process.

Ambivalence

Once the decision is made there are second thoughts. Even Susan, who wanted a baby very much, said "Are we sure we really want to do this? Oh, My God, we always thought about it, but this is a lot different" (S1). Christine talked about her fear. Was it the right decision? What about fatigue, the millions and millions of diapers, the losing of herself, the dependency, the vulnerability? What about her changing relationships? Will the baby be okay, be healthy? Work was manageable. How would she manage being a mother? In spite of these second thoughts, Christine said:

> I can't tell you how important it is for me to do this, in that I think it will make a difference in my life. You know there will be change and you

can't anticipate making that change. It diverges the course of your life forever. Men never truly have to deal with that, ever. (C1)

Even for those women who are open to a child in their life, the actual move to becoming mother takes time, time that at once is both immediate and gradual. It is immediate in the sense of "no turning back," and gradual in that the decision is made again and again with each new change. Still, at times, one wonders if it could be a mistake. Am I really ready? Do I not have some doubts? Am I not somewhat afraid?

Of course, for others who have taken diagnostic tests (such as amniocentesis) to detect fetal abnormality, the decision becomes even more difficult. The woman may have already experienced movement, and heard the heartbeat, and, now has to choose whether or not to accept this particular child in her life (Rapp 1984). There is a contradiction in the use of diagnostic ultrasound in pregnancy, the procedure makes the baby seem more real but holds the potential for the mother to keep the child at a distance in case there are problems (Hubbard 1984: 334).

The opening to the possibility of being mother, the creation of space in one's life for a child, begins with the thoughtful decision but is experienced by the pregnancy itself and, even further as we shall discuss later, by the arrival of the child. The decision, including both thought and action, is the beginning of the change. With the coming to a the decision about children in their lives, women begin their transformation to mothers.

Chapter 4

With Child: The Transformative Experience of the Presence of the Child

THE MEANING OF PRESENCE

T hough a woman may have chosen to conceive a child, she may not truly feel ready for the change that she expects is demanded of her. She may say, like Brenda, "It's too soon," "I'm not ready." Or like Christine, "Will I be able to cope?" Or Jane, "I haven't done enough. I want to establish a career." This occasional (or maybe persistent) ambivalence and doubt is exemplified by Jane's statement, "I thought maybe I was a little too young to have kids" (J3). Jane is thirty-two. Yet, it is Jane who puts into words a recognition of her move to mother through her own pregnancy. She said:

> Somewhere along the line the focus shifts. I can't pinpoint just when. I became less concerned about me and more concerned about the baby. The baby kicks and I can see the little appendages sticking out. That makes a difference. It is alive. It is real. I'm still apprehensive but not so ambivalent. (J2)

A woman does not make herself into mother—it happens through coexistence with the child. The presence of the child transforms.

> First, and foremost, the woman experiences her transformative character naturally and unreflectingly in pregnancy, in her relation to the growth of the child, and in childbearing. Here woman is the organ and instrument of the transformation of both her own structure and that of the child within her and outside her. Hence, for the woman the transformative character—even that of her own transformation—is from the beginning connected to the problem of the *thou* relationship . . . . Pregnancy is the second blood mystery . . . . The growth of the foetus already brings about a change of the woman's personality. (Neumann 1955: 31)

The being "with" child is not the "with" that means "as a companion," or "next-to," or "in the charge of." It could have those meanings, too, I suppose. However, being "with child" is a primordial relationship, peculiar to women who carry within their own bodies the body of another. It is a relationship that develops over time as the baby and the mother grow together. It is not simply a biochemical mix. Being "with child" is a commingling, an entangling, an interlacing that goes beyond companionship. It is a mysterious union, unlike any other. Not only is the fetus bound to the woman through the nourishing pathways running through the umbilical cord, but child and woman are truly one body. In spite of the separateness of their blood systems, the fetus cannot live without the oxygen and other nutrients which are provided through the remarkable capacities of the placenta. What affects the woman affects the fetus, and as the child evolves so does the mother. The mother and fetus are one, an indissoluble whole, yet two, a mother and a child. There is no closer union.

Thus, being *with child* moves a woman to motherhood in a unique, dramatic, and complex fashion. It is through her pregnant body that a woman comes to know herself as mother. There is no possibility for a woman to become a mother without a child, nor is it possible for a fetus to become a child without a woman. The presence of the child transforms a woman to mother. Through being "with" a woman a child is born. This does not mean a woman who adopts a child is not a mother. It is rather, that her experience of the child is different and therefore an adoptive woman's transformation to mother needs its own exploration and understanding.

The process in which men move to fatherhood, too, is different from women's move to motherhood. It can also be dramatic and powerful, but men who father will not experience the movement of the baby within. They do not feel the hiccups, the flips, the rolls, the startles of the developing child. They are not aware when the baby is still. It does not matter physically to the fetus how much their fathers drink (after conception). Men do not need to watch what they eat, nor do they experience enlarging and draining breasts. Nobody inquires about their weight, or wants to check their urine.

They do not have to wear a different set of clothes for several months. They know too that they miss out in something that is distinctive to women. Bill, Anna's husband, said, "There is always going to be something dear and special about a mother and child relationship—such a close knit thing. It is just something I can't hope to penetrate. A father's love is just going to be different" (A1). This "close-knit" relationship, made possible by conception, is for most women a life-long reality precisely because of its intimate inter-locking.

THE BODY "WITH CHILD"

"This *participation mystique* between mother and child is the original situation of container and contained" (Neumann 1955: 29). The archetype of the feminine describes the female body as a "real vessel" which holds containment as its elemental character (p. 44). Containment comes from Latin *tenēre* meaning "to hold together, to keep together, to maintain." It means to enclose. The female body encloses the developing child. The body-as-vessel image need not be a negative one, such as woman as an empty-vessel, or as a container for carrying the offspring of the man; but it can be a positive image that shows woman as the essential participant in the growth and development of the child.

> In the matriarchal world the woman as vessel is not made by man or out of man or used for his procreative purpose; rather the reverse is true: it is this vessel with its mysterious creative character that brings forth the male in itself and from out of itself. (Neumann 1955: 62)

The fact that a woman is the essential participant in the creation of the child needs to be clearly remembered and acknowledged. This is crucial in all aspects of the childbirth dialogue—whether in discussion of birthing or in the present controversial issue of abortion, and relinquishing and surrogate mothers.

Before conception there is no obvious space in a woman's body for the baby. The uterus is only inches big: and as a hollow, pear-shaped, muscular organ, its ability to house an eight-pound baby is unfathomable. For the first three months, the baby's presence is not obvious to anyone, perhaps not even to the woman herself. She may know the child is there while finding it difficult to actually imagine. She may start to feel different: heavy, tired, sometimes nauseated, with morning sickness, with breasts that tingle and become tender. As the fetus settles and grows, it pushes the uterus out into the larger abdominal cavity and crowds the other organs. Within, and as part of the woman's body, the baby begins to show itself to the world. So it is both the expanding body of the woman and the developing fetus, to-gether, that are creating the space for the baby.

Jane remarked about her realization of pregnancy. Her period was a week overdue. She was taking naps in the afternoon and her moods were very labile. She said, "I was not myself" (J1). Women wonder "just who they are." This is what Young calls a split subjectivity or a de-centered body subjectivity of "myself in the mode of not being myself" (1984: 48). The inner movements seem to belong to another, "another that is nevertheless my body." The normal bodily boundaries shift—one wonders where one's body begins and ends—the body's integrity is put into jeopardy. Brenda expresses surprise as she attempts to wear her winter coat from last year. In her mind's eye she holds the image of her pre-pregnant body, so that the way her clothes fit remind her that she is changing, remind her that she carries another being within. As Katherine finds it hard to move through a narrow space, she attempts to pull in her stomach—which, of course, no longer solves the problem. When looking in the mirror, Jane exclaimed, "Holy Smokes! Where does all that skin come from" (J2)! She is surprised at how she has grown. When the baby moves, the woman is reminded of her change; and when people respond to the baby first (glance first at her abdomen then her face), she may wonder "Who am I?" Or as Christine said, "Am I not a woman anymore" (C1)? Or Brenda, when treated "like she was going to break" said, "Leave me alone. I'm only pregnant, not a baby" (B1)!

Young calls this pregnant consciousness a double intentionality. There is a split between the tasks at hand. The one task is to have a baby, and the other, the awareness of the woman's own daily tasks and projects. "To be sure," Young said, "even in pregnancy there are times when I am so absorbed in my activity that I do not feel myself as body, but when I move or feel the look of another I am likely to be recalled to the thickness of my body" (1984: 51). When women hear the heartbeat, when the baby moves, or when the baby is seen through ultrasound examination, the true intention is evident (that is, to have a baby). Yet this intentionality, this felt presence of the baby, sometimes breaks down, and a woman may think, "Maybe I am just fat?" Susan wanted to be sure that others knew she was pregnant, "I kept saying to Paul, 'Do you think they can tell I'm pregnant?' " (S1). Anna, although she knew she was pregnant through her own calculations, by her slight morning sickness, through the doctor's examination, and through the positive pregnancy test, began to doubt. She said:

> Intellectually I *knew* but when I felt a kick that was pretty exciting. And then at 20 weeks I heard the heartbeat. The midwife acknowledged, "Yes, it is really there," which answered my question exactly. That was really an important day for me. (A1)

So Anna knew again of her pregnancy and the purpose of her changed body. A woman's knowledge of pregnancy and her transformation to mother is a process—a process that deepens her understanding of what she already knows (Polanyi 1969). It is a process of becoming what one already is.

Young points out that women's experience of their bodies in pregnancy is different than when one's body breaks down in illness and fatigue. As pregnant women we can "become aware of ourselves as body and take an interest in its sensations and limitations for their own sake experiencing them as a fullness rather than a lack" (1984: 50–1). Thus, the pregnant woman has the unique experience of being aware of her body as being *with* child while accomplishing her own tasks. "You just think twice about what you do," said Brenda (B1), "Before I would climb up all the boxes and pull down a forty-five pound box from the cooler. Now I think, 'Am I going to fall when I climb up there? Am I going to lose my balance? Will I get dizzy?' "

But this experience of accepting one's enlarged body, or of "thinking twice," may not necessarily be an easy one. It was not until Brenda's eighth month, in talking about her changing body, that she was able to say:

> Maybe I am getting used to my body. Now it doesn't seem so bad. When the baby moves you can see the ripple across your stomach. It seems like he or she is going to leave. That is why you are so big. It is not like you are just fat anymore. There is someone there. (B2)

Before that it was hard for her to accept "even if you understand it is a baby growing inside you—there are deposits of fat and stuff. It disgusts me—so far it is hard and firm but you know it will be jelly later on" (B1). The child's presence, through its movement, its reality as a separate person, allows Brenda to accept her own body, her body *with child* as her own. Others, also, experience their growing body as ugly. In a society that celebrates slimness it is not hard to understand the difficulty women have with accepting their growing bodies, especially when they have not yet truly experienced the presence of the child. But for Anna, Christine, and Katherine, it was easier. They enjoyed watching their tummies grow—feeling the hard roundness, appreciating their enlarged breasts. They enjoyed the presence of the child but they still wanted to look good, that is, not be seen as "frumpy"— nor did they want to hide their pregnancies. The body as vessel, for containment and nourishment of an other, transforms woman to mother.

Maternity Clothes

How does a woman clothe this transformed body? The move into maternity clothes is a public acknowledgment of the presence of the child. Before this outward affirmation, friends and acquaintances may wonder and speculate about the likelihood of pregnancy. But clothes tell the story. Especially in present society where women change to specific maternity clothes which tend to have a characteristic appearance. Katherine, Susan, and Anna talked about their efforts to find clothes that expressed their own individuality, and their own approach to accommodating their growing bodies. They said, for example:

Clothes have a tendency to deny the whole state of pregnancy because they have ruffles, and bows, and lace and everything else at the neck— to detract from your tummy. It seems they try to make me look like a virgin again. (A2)

Just bags. I'm not trying to hide my pregnancy but the clothes are just huge with puffed sleeves, and heavy-duty gather—which is baby-fying. I don't want to look like that, or to feel like that. (K1)

Like Susan, some of the other women were glad that they could sew so that they could wear the clothes in which they felt comfortable and that made them delighted with their growing bodies. None wanted to wear clothes that would reduce them to the childlike image that could even contain the suggestion of virginity. According to Brownmiller (1984: 81), "clothes make a statement. Clothes never shut up. They gabble on endlessly, making their intentional and unintentional points." How does the "statement" made by a woman's clothes affect her transformation to mother?

Chicago said, "Maternity clothes are obscene. They neuter the form and reality of the pregnant women by using inappropriate materials—little flowers, chintz, small plaids and checks—nothing to bring attention to the miracle and power of birth" (1985: 123). Anna's husband suggested that the ruffles, bows, and lace were used to help the pregnant woman feel more feminine, or, as Anna said earlier, to detract from the tummy (the growing child). Has femininity really been reduced to the "cutsie," the sweet, represented by the puffed sleeves that Anna, Katherine, and Susan did not want to exemplify? It is small wonder that women sometimes feel dependent on "experts" to guide their actions in pregnancy and in birth when they are encouraged in a "kind of infantilization" (Seiden 1978: 92) to which some maternity clothes contribute.

How much more in keeping with the power and miracle of the growing pregnant body is the fantasy of Chesler who wanted to wear a "hundred-breasted, thousand-jewelled garment of sapphire, a great coat of many colors. . . . Large, exotic clothes to loudly and gorgeously proclaim the miracle" . . . of her child's passage into being (1979: 33). Of course, Chesler acknowledged that such clothes cannot be found nor would there be any place to wear them—but her fantasy suggests the desire of women to express their own strength and the excitement and wonder at this time of intense and radical change that comes with the child's obvious presence.

Clothes that speak of the strength of femaleness, of femininity, and of the power to become a mother, support a woman's change in a powerful way. In a "society [that] often devalues and trivializes women, regards women as weak and dainty, the pregnant women can gain a certain sense of self-respect" (Young 1984: 52). Clothes that express a woman's own personality, neither denying her pregnancy nor her sexuality, help her to celebrate the wonderment of her bodily presence of the child, and assist her in the move to becoming a mother.

THE CHILD'S PRESENCE IN RELATIONSHIP

Toward the end of pregnancy women are tired of the big clothes and long to "get back into their jeans." There is a point when the presence of the child becomes a burden. Anna said:

> I think I've come to the point where I'm sick of being this huge. I don't get much sleep. I go to the bathroom every two hours. You've got your right side and your left side, can't sleep on your back. But I'm sure it is nature's way of getting me ready. (A3)

It almost feels that a woman no longer owns her body. The baby takes over and the woman merely goes along "unneeded by Nature's work" (Chesler 1979: 65). The difficult period of final waiting begins—the waiting for the actual child. The relationship with the baby starts in pregnancy. "The baby's movements within my body remind me to keep in touch," said Christine (C2). Jane, who thought that it may be easier to carry the baby inside rather than outside, begins to feel ready for the child "when I feel the active contractions my focus begins to shift to the thought of the actual child" (J2).

Touching the Baby

The women spoke of their relationship with the baby they carried—talking to him or her, touching, feeling the movement, noting the movement, sensing the rhythm. It was an intimate relationship that no one else shared. Christine said:

> Part of my relationship with the baby inside was the patting of myself, feeling him kick, responding to this kicking, and touching my abdomen. I felt really good about the shape, the hardness, and the roundness— loved rubbing cream on. It felt so good. (C4)

Other people too, sometimes want to feel the baby by touching the woman's tummy. At first the woman may feel confused, "What are you touching me for? How can I tell them I don't like it?" When the "toucher" was a male superior at work and when there wasn't much yet to show, Anna said, "I was not sure how to act" (A1). For Brenda it was, "they want to feel the baby kicking which really embarrasses me. Like it is too personal" (B1). Of course, if it is someone close to you, "It is terrific," said Anna. "My mother is coming for a visit and says that she wants to come to feel my tummy" (A1). Katherine's statement shows the paradox of this experience, "I don't think they were patting my stomach even though it was my stomach they were patting" (K1). The body being touched is one's own, yet it is the baby that is being touched.

Touching of a woman's body, as baby, again shows the remarkable and unique experience of pregnancy—being another while being oneself. As the baby grows bigger there is less confusion. It is more obvious to the woman herself, and the person who reaches toward the woman/child, just who is being touched. Towards the end of pregnancy it may be that one loves to have people touch one's baby who is now so obviously present. Bill, Anna's husband, talked about the attraction of the pregnant woman's tummy, "I can understand it, because it is almost irresistible. To feel her tummy is just great. I feel my sister's tummy too and it feels different. I can understand why men do it. It draws me to it—it is a fascination" (A1). There is something about the roundness of the pregnant belly that invites touching. Is it like the soft smoothness of the baby's cheek or the intrigue of the lover's face? The desire to touch the woman's tummy to feel its firmness, roundness, and the movement of the baby is perhaps the recognition of the mysterious presence of the baby within the woman. "The inside maybe is the baby but the outside is me," said Susan (S3).

Touching the Woman

Although the women did not readily speak about their experience of sex during pregnancy, Christine described the changed relationship with her husband. "It is still good," she said. When she asked him if it was different for him, he admitted that it was, "I just feel different about what the vagina is for and what the breasts are for" (C1). It makes one understand that women's bodies are made to accommodate a child, and the child's presence makes that obvious. A pregnant woman's body has a different kind of richness, perhaps "awe-inspiring," which according to Barber and Skaggs (1975) is a "primitive signal perhaps reaching back to the beginnings of human life." Bill said of Anna, "I thought she was radiant before, you know (honestly), but since she has become pregnant I can't take my eyes off her. There is a radiance about her that I'm fascinated by" (A1). This fascination may be an acknowledgment of something holy—a reverence for life. It may also be a confusion about the whole sexual nature of the childbirth for women.

> Before you were pregnant nobody talked about sex or anything like that. But once you are pregnant the taboos all go away, everyone knows you've done it so it must be legitimate to talk about it. It is really weird. (J1)
> All of a sudden they found that you're pregnant, and my goodness, you can't hear this joke. All of sudden you've regained your chastity and you're Miss Innocence. Maybe they think the baby can hear. (S3)

Is this confusion an expression of the separation of sexuality and pregnancy? Niles Newton, psychologist and early (in the 1950s) supporter of breastfeeding, notes that in the female reproductive triad of coitus, birth, and lactation, there is a tendency in our society to place special emphasis on the first . . . and ignore the sexual aspects of the latter two" (Seiden 1978: 91). In the "awe" of the woman with child, there is a danger of ignoring or downplaying the sexual nature of this experience for women. In a society that sometimes discourages female sexuality, as well as assertiveness and aggressiveness, one is not sure how to act in the presence of the pregnant woman.

Feeling Vulnerable

"There are these guys in the office, very old-fashioned, who when I come into the office—it is like, 'You'd better sit down,' sort of like I am crippled or something" (C1). At first it seems strange but as the pregnancy progresses women experience a changed sense of themselves and their need for others. They begin to feel vulnerable and more willing to accept the attentive support that is offered them through much of their pregnancy. Christine said:

> I have felt more dependent than I have ever felt in my life. I feel physically vulnerable, that is, if I am with a bunch of people in a crowd, I could easily be thrown off balance. Through the winter, especially, when I am driving the car, I don't want these crazy drivers coming near me. It is just that there is a baby here! Just lately, in the last three weeks, I feel careful about what I lift and haul and carry. Before it would be hard for me to let someone else do it. I mean, I am very strong and feel very strong and very capable and "I can do this!" (C2)

A woman may experience others as considerate and protective: colleagues who leave a parking space next to the door, fellow workers who lift heavy boxes, racquetball partners who no longer want to play, or a father who think his daughter is working too hard. Since the woman feels more vulnerable, she is therefore more accepting of offers of assistance. Earlier in pregnancy the woman may often have resisted or even resented offers of help, late in pregnancy she tends to be appreciative. It is not just the fact of a large and awkward body, there is an attitude change that has to do with the relationship of mother and child. "I'm careful when I cross the road now—before I just charged across. I've changed, and Nathan has responded to the change. He is protective of me because of the presence of the baby" (C1). To protect the relationship with her child, the woman accepts her vulnerability and need for others. "I think it is kind of preparing me for the fact that when the baby comes I am not going to raise it by myself. I am going to need help," said Anna (A2).

But again, as with all human experience, the sense of vulnerability and the need for protectiveness is more complicated. Anna's and Brenda's husbands expressed a desire to lessen their wife's anguish (A1, B2) Anna stated that such sentiments are misplaced and that the desire to protect may have gone too far.

> You see, I don't think that protectiveness is necessarily a valid feeling . . . because women are built for this situation. The body takes care. The body does it all. We don't need episiotomies, we don't need enemas, we don't need to be shaved. Our body takes care of it. (A1)

Brenda, too, reacts when Tom makes decisions for her such as ordering milk instead of coffee at lunch, and when he wants her to have a cesarean birth because he sees it as more humane. Women are beginning to identify, for themselves, the way in which protectiveness is appropriate or not. Being supportive of the vulnerability that occurs with the presence of child, while fostering the woman's own sense of self as a capable and responsible woman, can help rather than hinder a woman's transformation to mother. Anna and Christine, both very independent women, spoke at some length about their need for a sharing relationship in the project of parenting. They felt the experience of carrying and giving birth had helped them to realize and accept their need for others.

THE TEMPORAL DUE DATE

"What is your due date?" "When are you expecting?" are questions repeatedly asked of a pregnant woman. Such questions are suggestive that the childbirth process is for the child, that the woman's task is nothing but to watch and wait. In one sense, this is true. That is, pregnancy ends. The child is born. But in terms of a woman's transformation to mother, the "due" date is just one moment in a larger endeavor. The temporality of the move to motherhood cannot be limited to such a linear time frame as "waiting" during pregnancy. The woman is not merely waiting. She is moving, growing, and changing (Young 1984). Throughout pregnancy she experiences herself as source and participant in a creative process. "Though she does not plan or direct it, neither does she let it merely wash over her; rather, she *is* the process, this change" (Young 1984: 54). So not only does time stretch out toward a "due" date but the moments and days take on a depth that reaches into her very self, her body—and transforms her. Anna put it this way:

> The birth itself is one event on a continuum, not an end in itself. I think it has to be that way. The gestation period is nine months, and I think that with every month and every week you are able to go further and further beyond the birth. I mean you are focusing on the birth date—the birthday—but for me the further along that I am pregnant, the more I am able to see beyond that. (A2)

Could it be that the pervasive search for the actual date of the child's birthday overlooks the growth process that a woman experiences? Does the focus on the due date overlook the day-to-day growth and development of the mother herself?

The pregnant woman is called expectant, an attitude of excitement and wonder. She prepares herself for the birth—she prepares herself to be mother. As she focuses on "zero day," as Anna said, she also waits for herself to become a mother. Katherine (K2), eight months pregnant, said she did not feel like a mother, "Maybe it happens when you have a child, and have worked out things with your child." Yet, in the next breath she described a change that she noticed in herself, "The other day at the doctor's office, when I held a little (two weeks old) sleeping baby on my chest, I felt kind of choked up, a little bit, kind of teary with a baby that small." She was being opened to the possibility of herself as mother by the actual life she carried below her heart. She expects she will feel like a mother when the baby comes, without realizing the gradual evolution of her expectancy.

The focus of attention on the "due day," or the Expected Date of Confinement, may be a form of waiting that is found in the world of instrument-machinery (Fujita 1985). Such an instrumental, means-ends, type of waiting can be contrasted with waiting "in the natural world," or waiting "in the world of becoming." Waiting in the natural world involves trust in the power and process of nature which are independent of human operations and attitudes. Waiting in the world of becoming, which is "becoming ourselves, becoming more human," or maybe, "becoming a mother," involves a dialectic between "how we wait" and "what is waited for." "In the world of becoming, we can even say that the very ways of 'how we wait' enable us to be aware of what has been out of our reach and, thus, enriches, and transforms the initial 'what we waited for' " (Fujita 1985: 113). Attention to the experience of the woman herself during pregnancy attunes one to the very real growth and change that occur for women during their experience of waiting for the child.

THE PRESENCE OF THE CHILD TRANSFORMS SPACE

Maybe I can talk about how I feel about the world. I'm more intro-spective—catch myself daydreaming at work, and just thinking about the miracle of creating a life. What is going on inside is wonderful—I have more concern about mankind and justice. (A1)

The pregnant woman notices that the world is full of pregnant women, mothers, and babies. When I said to Katherine that I had not noticed many pregnant women, she did not believe me. "Oh, come on!" she said, "There is a baby boom. It is incredible" (K1). Others, like Jane, said they watched the interaction between mothers and babies. They noticed what they eat and drink, whether the mothers smoke, what they do, and what they say to their children. They want to know how one lives, as mother, in the world.

And the "world" noticed them too.

If you go into a crowded place, a lot of people stop and look at you and smile at you. Whereas before you would just walk in. . . . We went into the lounge for a drink, and I find that people really make you feel uneasy, like you are doing something terrible, and you are only drinking orange juice. Like "come on!" (B1)

Saturday night was our Christmas party. I was drinking orange juice, good healthy stuff. . . . When I get up to dance everybody around you, "Careful, Mom!, Should you be dancing, Mom?" It is just, "Oh, I'm pregnant, I should sit in my corner." (B2)

It feels a little odd to be pregnant and sitting in a bar. It really does. (K1)

It is confusing. With the presence of the child in her body, a woman sees the world as changed and experiences that changed world in various ways. Brenda, as we heard, did not want be seen differently—she wanted to be just herself. Katherine, on the other hand, saw herself as changed, and began to question her actions. Both begin to question what is appropriate behavior for a woman with child? Maybe pregnancy is a time when women are "exercised" into motherhood as suggested by van Manen (1986a). Women begin to learn how to act in the world as mothers.

Chapter 5

Separation: The Transformative Experience of Birthing Pain[1]

CAN BIRTHING PAIN HAVE MEANING?

M any women seem to want to prepare for the actual birth experience. They do so by attending childbirth classes, by reading the ever-growing supply of childbirth books (many of which are now written by women who have been through the childbirth experience themselves), and by talking to friends and colleagues, doctors and nurses, and others. In the preparation and anticipation of birth, women are surrounded by thoughts of the pain that they will experience. I recall that after teaching childbirth classes for a number of years I was asked by a woman from one of these classes, who had had a long and difficult labor, "Why didn't you tell me about the pain?" I was taken aback because I thought I had. But how does one talk about the pain of childbirth? It is usually the aspect of pain that surfaces in the horror stories. It is the pain that one is said to forget over time. With labor inevitably comes pain for most women, and it is the pain that is thought about during pregnancy:

Now I'm starting to question and wonder about my ability to handle the birth thing—that whole process without drugs—and though I'm committed to that whole idea, will I be able to handle it? (A2)

I figure it is going to hurt so why worry. It is going to happen. It is not going to hurt for 15 years, just a day or so—not like an illness. (B1)

I'm not worried about the labor and delivery really. If for no other reason than that thousands of women do it—and it is for a short time. (J2)

I'm waiting to compare labor pain to a headache. I have headaches that last for a day and a half, maybe two days—and I can stand that. (S3)

The pain comes from the experience of separation of mother and child—physically generated by the tumultuous rhythm of the contractions which open the cervix to allow the passage of the baby down the birth canal and thrust the baby into life as a separate being. The pain is also the splitting of the unique and particular unity of the mother and child exemplified by "the presence of the child." According to Rich, "the pains of labor have a peculiar centrality for women, and women's relationship—both as mothers and simply as female beings—to other kinds of painful experience" (1976: 15).

Throughout pregnancy Susan talked of not trusting her body, she talked about her eating habits, her clothes, her aches and pains, and she talked about her vulnerability. It seems that her body was experienced as separate, as disembodied from her being. Even her baby was not a part of her. "It's sort of somebody down there, but not an extension of myself" (S3). Yet after the birth Susan talked about how the labor, and the pain, had brought her and her husband closer together, and how she, too, seemed to become more integrated and whole. She related the painfulness of this experience to other painful experiences in her life, her mother's illness, and the breakup of her first marriage. It seems that the pain may be one experience that contributes to a woman's transformation such that Susan could say, "I look back and can't believe how I used to be. I can't recognize who I was" (B3).

One has to wonder if there is something important in the pangs of childbirth that is true for all women, those who pleasure in its labor, those who endure, and those who suffer. Some births are short and intense, some long and exhausting, and some need medical intervention and treatment with forceps, medication, and cesarean delivery. Christine experienced intense, excruciating pain (partly due to the use of forceps) and yet two months later said, "I'm glad I didn't miss it and I would wish other women could experience it." Then she paused and wondered, "Why did I say that?," and goes on:

I don't think one should focus on the pain, that women should have to experience pain. But in the pain there is an experience of being inward and involved in feeling the pain—not enjoying it but taking hold, enduring, or whatever you do to handle it—and knowing that it is going to produce a child. That is what it is, not to focus on the pain, but to see what the pain does to you, how it changes you. (C4)

Is it possible that the separation, and its accompanying pain, is a penetrating aspect of a woman's transformation? What can birthing pain show us about a woman's transformation to mother?

Letting Go Assumptions

In order to explore the nature of birthing pain, it is important to let go, for a moment at least, of some of our current assumptions and beliefs. These may include ideas that:

Pain should be denied. Some childbirth educators have thought that by removing the word "pain" from the language of birthing, they will prepare women to take a more positive posture and to accept more readily the challenge and joy of the birth. Some talk of "contractions," others refer to "rushes," or "discomfort" to mean the experienced pain. Anna said:

> Early in pregnancy I had felt that I am not going to see this as a painful experience, I'm going to relax, and go with the flow, but after having listened to a tape of a woman in labor, and hearing about transition, and how disorientated you become—a very tough time—really dispelled any notions that there would be no pain. . . . Pain really does exist. (A2)

While a woman's positive attitude is important, denial of pain may create expectations not borne out in reality. What is being denied in the denial of birthing pain?

Pain must be relieved. The belief that pain must be relieved pervades our society, from the advertisement of over-the-counter drugs to the medical need to "give something for the pain." Although human suffering must be prevented or reduced, let us stand back from the expectation that relief or removal of the pain of childbirth is a primary and necessary goal. Rich (1976: 152) suggested that this notion "is a dangerous mechanism, which can cause us to lose touch not just with our painful sensations but with ourselves." Could it be that the fear and anxiety of pain stands in the way of drawing on the fundamental source of life and spirit women have? Fear of the pain may be a result of tales, anecdotes, literature, and medical approaches to childbirth. Until recently, the written texts about birth came from the hands and minds of men who had observed and described but had not experienced. The knowledge and the support that was originally available to women, from mother to daughter, from midwife to laboring woman, from older to younger, is once more becoming available. The reclaiming of the childbirth experience by women has done much to dispel untruths and has reaffirmed women at the center of birthing practices. Birthing is their experience. As women accept their bodies, their bigness, their appetites, and their feelings as well as their intellect, they will regain their sense of power. Rich (1976: 292) said, "we need to imagine a world in which every woman is the presiding genius of her own body. . . . Then women will truly create new life." What is taken away in attempting to take away the pain of giving birth?

Pain is only negative. Childbirth pain is a normal accompaniment of birthing and may arise from dilation of the cervix, the contraction and distension of the uterus, distension of the outlet, vulva, and perineum, and from factors such as pressure on the bladder, rectum and other pain-sensitive structures in the pelvis (Bonica 1975, 1984). Birthing pain brings life. The fact that childbirth is now primarily a medical event, occurring in an atmosphere associated with sickness and death, supports the underlying notion that the pregnancy-birth event is a disease condition. In a nursing text on pain (Meinhardt and McCaffery 1983), labor pain is included in the chapter on pain syndromes along with phantom limb pain, trigeminal neuralgia, arthritis, headache, and pain syndromes associated with cancer. In fact, the term "syndrome" is defined as a "a group of signs and symptoms that collectively indicate or characterize disease, psychological disorder, or other abnormal conditions" (Morris 1978: 1305).

Of course, there is a danger in romanticizing pain. We know childbirth and its pain has taken its toll, with death and horror so vividly described in medical case histories as well as biographies and novels. It is small wonder that women have welcomed prescribed anesthesia, believing it would mean less pain and danger at birth (Hubbard 1984: 338). At one level pain is a sign of distress and possible danger; yet birthing pain can be normal, and with the pain comes life. Can birthing pain be shown to be a positive normal experience?

Pain is punishment. The word pain derives from the Greek *poinē* meaning penalty. This origin is suggestive of the notion that women are being punished for the "crime" of pregnancy, or symbolically, for tasting of the tree of knowledge, that is, "knowing too much" (Seiden 1978: 95). Is it possible that nonacceptance of the pain, or the fear of pain, comes from women's nonacceptance of or alienation from their bodies, leading to fear of helplessness, fear of dependence, and fear of inappropriate behavior? Rather than accepting the notion that childbirth pain is a punishment to be mutely accepted, one wonders if women could be seen to acknowledge their physicalness, their passion, their sexuality, their whole female existence, childbirth pain may be approached as a challenge and opportunity. Yet even here there are limits between ennobling pain and self-destructive hurtful pain. But can giving birth be an event of proud endurance of pain in the service of a desired goal, not unlike contact and endurance sports (Seiden 1978: 101)? Can birthing pain be seen as an opportunity and a challenge?

Pain can be explained. There are theories that explain childbirth pain physically, psychologically, sociologically, and culturally. These theories and explanations contribute to our understanding of pain, but they also fragment the sense of wholeness of the pain experience. When we explain, we stand apart from the phenomenon and observe, trying to fit everything into systematic order thus belying the mystery (Olson 1986) and women's participation in that mystery. Exploring the phenomenon of birthing pain is an attempt to grasp that primordial wholeness of the experienced pain—the participation of women in their pain. Is there experiential wholeness within the nature of women's birthing pain?

Can Birthing Pain be Described?

Birthing pain, like other pain, is difficult to describe. "Its resistance to language is not simply one of its incidental or accidental attributes but is essential to what it is," said Scarry (1985). "This resistance to language is because physical pain, unlike any other state of consciousness—has no referential content. It is not *of* or *for* anything" (p. 5). But here we need to look again. The pain of childbirth *is* different from the enveloping effects of other pain: "these pains one could follow with one's mind" (Margaret Mead, in Sorel 1984: 339). And birthing pain produces a child. However violent and terrible the pains are, this connection needs to be remembered: "I reached down and took him out . . . put him on my belly . . . I couldn't take my eyes off him" (V). Or as Susan said, "You get a prize in the end. You've accomplished something that you can look back and say, 'Gee, I did that' " (S3). Thus, what is at stake is the meaning of the childbirth pain, so more than just the physical sensations of the pain needs to be taken into consideration. If birthing pain is likened to the pain of mountain climbing, the pain of running the last few yards of an Olympic race, the pain of the downhill skier in search of the gold medal, rather than the pain of arthritis, cancer, or other illness (Melzack, Taenzer, Feldman, and Kinch 1980), would that change women's preparation for and attitude about the pain?

> I use the analogy all the time—bicycling. We just telephoned a friend this morning who was on our cycling trip with us and I said, "Dave, you know, when I'm in labor and doing all that hard work, I'm going to be thinking about going over that mountain . . . I was reduced to tears [on that trip] because of my frustration, and because I couldn't breathe . . . but I mean, I did it . . . I made it on my own power. (A2)

If childbirth pain was embraced as part of the mastery of a worthwhile activity, it may not be thought of as hardship (Kittay 1983: 124). Childbirth pain is *of* and *for* the child, and in this fact is contained the possibility of personal good, "I did that," or as Paula said, "I can do anything now" (P1).

But still it is hard to find the right words. Women say the pain is powerful, intense, overwhelming, cramp-like, stretching, burning, pressuring, tiring, and exhausting. They say:

I withdrew into myself, had few thoughts. (H)
I was immersed in a physical sensation, lost awareness of time and what was going on around me. (V)
I feared that I wouldn't be able to stand the pain—would lose control of myself—maybe even die. (P)
I was brought to the core of myself. I was pitted against myself. (H)
It was definitely, definitely painful. When she crowned, it hurt a lot. I can't deny that. But as each hour passes the memory gets less pronounced. And look what I have to show for it. . . . [seven months later] I've almost forgotten—am surprised how easy it was. (A4, A6)
I have a picture in my mind's eye of being in pain, but I can't remember the pain. (J3)
After the birth I almost had a feeling that perhaps I imagined the pain. Was it really as hard as I thought it was? (P2)

"Who can remember pain once it is over?" wrote Atwood, "All that remains of it is a shadow, not in the mind even, in the flesh. Pain marks you, but too deep to see" (1985: 135).

I AM MY PAINFUL BODY

I had my first contraction in the bathroom. It came from nowhere—an internal tornado picked up and hurled every organ toward my skin but nothing showed outwardly; the force was wholly absorbed. I couldn't recognize my own body in pain. I endured two before the words came to me: I am in labor. (Israeloff 1982: 86–7)

Childbirth pain is something deep and powerful: "It is different than [other pain] I've ever experienced—low back pain—deep pubic pain" (V). True, there is the localized, surface pain, such as the burning and stinging as the tissue stretches to release the baby's head, but at the same time, there is that deep inner pain which expresses itself as "being in pain."

The inwardness of childbirth pain is experienced by the feeling of un-reality, of being in a fog. Or a sense that time has stopped, is going on forever, is irrelevant. There is little awareness of the people around. "I don't remember what was talked about. I was totally inward" (I). The origin of the word "birth," from the Old Norse *burdhr* or *bher*, means to carry, to bear children. The carrying, the holding of the child, the woman-body-vessel (Neumann 1955) is the nature of woman's body. As a woman, I *am* this body, I *am* this pain. Birth, *bher*, also refers to bearing as an enduring. To bear, to carry on, to endure the pain is a part of the birth experience.

Pain is experienced by one's stance in relation to it—as a woman of autonomy and personal power or as a woman at the mercy of the environment or the doctor, alienated from her body and subject to fearful thoughts and imaginings. As women accept and take hold of their power, to figuratively and literally "stand up" and actively birth their own children rather than be delivered, as in the vulnerable "lying on one's back" position, they do not deny the pain but carry it. The pain-as-experienced is empowered by their way of standing in relationship to it: their riding with it and enduring it, or their being overwhelmed by it. Both enduring and suffering are experienced by women.

> Something was amiss, the next contraction on its way. Assuming that I was in the first stage of labor, I began the appropriate breathing tech-nique—carefully paced inhalations followed by gently blown exhalations. It worked in the sense that without it I'd have been swallowed by the pain and with it I could contend. But I had never been less distracted in my life. Nothing else was in my universe but the pain. (Israeloff 1982: 86)

In the attention to the pain there is a realization that the pain is not static and unchanging but something dynamic and moving, and the power of attention can become a key factor in working with the pain and lessening the pain. By focusing attention inward, we can gain a better understanding of the numerous signals our bodies transmit regarding what to do to help ourselves through the pain (Heckler 1984: 61). The body has wisdom of its own which does not lie (Woodman 1985) but perhaps needs time to find its own rhythm. The universal acceptance of Cartesian philosophy, which sep-arates mind and locates self-hood with the "thinking thing," *res cogitans*, has invaded our thought to such an extent that there is danger that we have lost touch with that body wisdom, the "material being," *res extensa*. In childbirth pain embodiment—understood in the notion "I am my body"—becomes a concrete reality not to be ignored. Merleau-Ponty reminds us that it is our bodily presence in the world that makes knowing possible: through our body we speak to the world—because the world in turn speaks to us through our body (Martel and Peterat 1985).

Yet the regular, intense, continuous contractions take their toll of energy and resources. Exhausted with the pain of fatigue, the feeling is one of "I just cannot go on." "Too tired to say anything, I push with all my might. I'm the Lilliputian. I may not be able to do it. It's beyond me to give birth to you" (Chesler 1979: 115). The work, exertion, effort, is not just the physical power of the uterus, nor is it just the intellectual power of the mind, but the unity of self which calls women to use all their resources. Women carry on, especially if aware that the baby is soon to be born. Of course, there is no other option. "There is no turning back, you are in it. The only choice is your attitude about it. With a good attitude it is so much better" said Anna's sister about her own thirty-six hour labor (A4).

The pain of labor demands action. Grunting, screaming, walking, finding a comfortable position, active relaxation, breathing patterns, focusing atten-tion, or having a bath. Any of these may free women from the state of passive suffering. Women have said things like: "I didn't know what to do and needed someone to help me" (X); "I tried to find a comfortable position, was impatient, angry, and shaking" (F); or "I screamed, or wanted to scream, to bite on something. I cried because it hurt so much" (E). We need to ask, "What can be done?"

The Cry of Pain

"I will cry out like a woman in travail. I will gasp and pant" (Isaiah 42:14). The Australian myth of Eingana (the Great Earth Mother, fertility herself, the source of all life, all forms of being) gives a clue to this cry:

> Eingana's travail to give birth is also the explanation of the sound made by the "bull-roarer" in the Kunapappi ritual . . . . Eingana was rolling about, every way, on the ground. She was groaning and calling out . . . making a big noise. (Meltzer 1981: 11)

A big noise! "The noise came from where? My depths for sure. It amazed me. The bull's roar—a perfect description for what it felt like and sounded to me" (P2). Anna, too, talked about the "primal, guttural kind of noise that came when pushing, and the whinnying noise while crowning. Making the noise helped the effort it seemed" (A4).

> These cries amazed me. With my first child, I hadn't felt any desire to scream or cry. Now I had the impression that I was rousing the entire hospital. Never in my life had I wailed like that before. It was as if the cries didn't belong to me. . . . At one point I heard myself crying out in a different way: long, trembling howls, like the cries of a baby. I realize now that these cries protected me, not from the pain, but from a traumatic inscription of this pain on my psyche. It was a kind of catharsis; by screaming, I let the pain leave my body. (quoted in Odent 1984a: 55)

Earlier in labor there may be moments of laughing. I recall Paula. There were times during the long day of labor when the house rang with her boisterous laughter. Perhaps it was as we manipulated her laboring body through the awkward space to have her sink into a tub of warm, soothing water, or maybe it was when some funny incident triggered a hooting guffaw. "Laughing felt good," she said later. Jane, too, was surprised at the fun her sister-in-law had in early labor:

> They were giggling and laughing, counting contractions and having a great time. Finally they left for the hospital at 1:30 A.M. Melissa was having some discomfort, but not obvious pain. She was able to joke through it. (J2)

Crying, laughing, the bull's roar, the screams, the whinnying, all express the woman's experience of the pain and the intensity of labor. She may not even be entirely conscious that the sound is coming from herself (Barber and Skaggs 1975: 39).

Giving voice to women's pain, the pain of childbirth, assists women's use of the pain experience to express themselves and the reality of their world. It transforms women's experience of pain to something useful to them.

> Near the end of my labor, I began to curse. I can't remember what I said: I had lost control of my senses. That experience has outlived the actual moment of birth. To think that I could act like this in front of other people! Yet it was as if, after losing my own voice for so many years, I had finally found it again. (quoted in Odent 1984a: 55)

Nonetheless, pain should not be stoically endured by women for some psychological or physiological value (Meinhardt and McCaffery 1983: 237). By giving voice to pain, women may help themselves through it. Women can use the pain to express themselves rather than let the pain defeat them, belittle them, or leave them feeling helpless and angry.

Finding a Position

In 1884, the doctor Engelmann, in an ethnographic account of laboring women from various cultures wrote, "the parturient must be guided by her own actions, and in a position assumed by her own comfort and by the dictates of her instinct . . . . The recumbent position retards labor and is inimical to easy, safe, and rapid delivery" (p. 149). Odent, another doctor, nearly a hundred years later (1981), after the recumbent position had been used almost routinely by obstetricians, hearkens back to the instinctual knowledge of the body.

> These last years, we understand better and better what to do to help the mother become more instinctive, to forget what is cultural, to reduce the control of the neocortex, to change her level of consciousness so that the labor seems to be easier. (Odent 1981: 9)

If women obey their own impulses and become more instinctual, they may assume a squatting, kneeling, or sitting posture. According to Engelmann (1884), "this would . . . often do away with the necessity of resorting to the forceps, which, though a great blessing, too often become the reverse in the hands of eager obstetricians, who are inclined to use them on the least occasion, or without any real occasion at all" (p. 149).

How does the birthing posture affect birthing pain and women's understanding of themselves? Susan found that sitting or standing was much easier, in spite of the availability of the costly solid oak bed[2] in her hospital birthing room. Christine had discussed the best position for labor with her doctor before the birth. He had said, "You should squat when you deliver, you shouldn't sit [referring to the birthing chair]. There is a difference, because the birth canal is not straight down, it's curved. So you need to squat" (C3). But in her labor, Christine had only two choices, the delivery table or the birthing chair. Later when Christine discussed it with me, she said that she needed to say to her doctor, "If squatting is the way, how come you are not doing it?" And then she said, "Of course, they are not set up to handle it. You have to have someone to assist you, and they can't cope with that in hospital. So I presume that is why he doesn't do it. I should ask him" (C3).

Many hospitals allow only one support person to attend the laboring woman and do not have enough staff around to give the squatting woman the constant attention she needs. At home it was different as Anna described:

> Anyway, when I wanted to push, I tried in a forty-five degree angle sitting up, and that didn't seem to work and then Bill helped me get into a squatting position. I found that really good, and I had no trouble pushing—a very primal feeling. Betty [a friend] and Mary [mother-in-law] came and got on either side of me and I could just kind of lean on them. (A4)

Finding a good position helps the woman to deal with the pain. Christine, who just recently had her second child found that this time she stood by the bed most of the time, enduring the contractions by slow controlled breathing, leaning on her hands, and slowly rocking her body through the pain. She was inward—her husband sat on a chair beside her. She did it herself and said, "It was wonderful" (Christine, Personal Communication, March 2, 1986).

SPACE FOR PAIN

There is not much tolerance for pain in everyday life. We try to remove pain as quickly as we can with drugs, with entertainment, with sex, with divorce, or with technology. Anna said:

> I don't think society allows us to deal with the harsher realities of life, and I don't think we are better off for it. . . . What we lose is the intensity of living—a vitality, the risk of being hurt or the risk of the responsibility of friendship and all that is involved in that. (A3)

But surely life should not be harsher. Surely, we have enough pain. Christine, Anna, Susan, Paula, and Jane described how the pain of birthing was important to their own personal growth, but, of course, they did not want to suffer pain unnecessarily. Is there pain that is necessary? If so, how can one experience necessary pain so that it is an opportunity for growth and change? How can pain serve the process of transformation rather than debilitate or cause "residual maternal and psychological problems" which, according to Meinhardt and McCaffery (1983: 37), result from severe pain?

How can the space in which women give birth aid them to transform their experience of pain into something useful for their lives?

One woman said, "The pain is powerful, overwhelming. I feared that I couldn't handle it. My anxieties related to how I would perform" (E). Susan, as well as Christine and Jane, wanted to be "good." "I was really worried that I was being really noisy. I didn't want to be yelling, and then it's hard to judge how loud you are" (S4). To be good means not to "make too much noise." It means to be "cooperative if one doesn't feel cooperative," and to not "make a scene." In their effort to be good, to please hospital staff, do women not fit to some predesigned criteria of what is appropriate behavior? In their effort to "be good," do women not deny the potential they have to help themselves through the pain?

Being "At Home"

Susan and Jane gave birth in the birthing room, the new hospital structure which has been designed to humanize obstetrical care by providing a more comfortable environment. The birthing room concept allows for the woman to labor and deliver in the same room as opposed to moving from one room to another at the beginning of the birth itself. The birthing room is generally furnished with curtains, carpets, an easy chair, coffee table, telephone, television, and a bed. In this setting "parents are provided with the opportunity to discuss their preferences in relation to medication, treatments and potential intervention and become partners, with the nursing and medical staff, in the decision-making process" (Field, Campbell, and Buchan 1985: 1–2). In the study by Field et al., parents indicated that what was satisfying about being in the birthing room was the privacy and the sense of control of their own birth experience (p. 137). They also found it comfortable, home-like, restful and helpful for relaxation. One often hears the term "home-like" in reference to the birthing room. Home-like is generally associated with the wallpaper, the rugs, and the softer decor. In spite of the obvious benefits that have resulted from the introduction of the birthing rooms, it is important to ask a deeper question about what the notion of a home-like environment has to do with the problem of childbirth pain? How does the environment of the birthing room affect a woman's experience of pain? How does it help her transformation to mother?

Do not the carpeted floor, the piped-in music, the bedside television, the handy telephone, sound more like a motel than a home? One then wonders whose home the home-like birthing room is like—the doctor's, the nurse's, the birthing woman's, or the traveler's? An exploration of the nature of "at homeness" (Baldursson 1985) may be helpful. The Oxford English Dictionary (1971) defines home as "a dwelling place, one's proper abode; the place of one's dwelling and nurturing and the feelings associated with it; a place where one properly belongs, etc." (pp. 349–51). To be at home, is "to be at ease—in one's element, unconstrained and unembarrassed, familiar with things; accessible to callers; and so on." Do we not invite our guests "to make themselves at home," to be at ease, to be comfortable? We know the times we are "at home" in other people's home and when we are not. What is it that makes one feel at home? What does it mean to feel at home in a hospital?

Being oneself. To be at home is to be ourselves (Buckley 1971, quoted in Baldursson 1985). To "be ourselves" requires no explanations, no guard against the misconceptions of others, no playing of "games," and no fear of abandonment. In such an environment, one does not worry about being good—in fact, one does not even think about the need to be good. Of course, one thinks about being kind and considerate, but "being good" is usually an attribute parents value in children. At home we are who we truly are. We leave behind our public roles—as hairdresser, lawyer, professor, office worker. We usually take off our work clothes, and get into our jeans—and we relate to our home mates as lover, friend, companion, or husband. We put our feet up, we have a bath, prepare meals, shave our legs, or make love. We do not need to excuse ourselves. Here we are at home.

Christine said, "I can remember complaining that I didn't want to co-operate" (C3). Perhaps the question needs to be asked, what did it mean for Christine to feel that she needed to cooperate? If the woman is "at home" where she is the center of the action, the central figure in the act of birthing her child, then the people surrounding her would need to be cooperating with her. The word "cooperate" tells us again that Christine deeply felt that she was dependent on others to make the various decisions with which she would need to cooperate. In a sense, then, one could think that Christine was not "at home"—was not being herself. Her resistance to what was done to her was expressed by a desire to "not cooperate" rather than do the things the way she wanted. "Unless the woman has some psychiatric disorder impairing her competence for decision making . . . she should have, as nearly as possible, the same degree of control over her activities and companions as she has in her own home" (Seiden 1978: 101). Being in her own home, Paula said, "I feel I rode the contractions in the sense of expressing what they felt like to me at the time—felt comfortable about being spontaneous in both vocal and physical reactions—being home felt right" (P2). She did what was right for her, her companions cooperated with her. Anna, because she had not had the "cleansing" enema, had to deal with the problem of "kind of pushing at both ends," which she described as her most embarrassing experience. "I felt kind of bad about that, but the midwives were really discreet about it" (A4). In the privacy of her own home, she did not feel rejected or frowned upon—just momentarily embarrassed.

Having one's things. "Have you packed your bag?" There are lists of things that the woman should take to hospital to make her stay more comfortable. Essential materials are provided but she wants to bring her own things. During labor, however, personal things are put away. The hospital garb is provided which helps the woman to fit into the patient role. The cups, the linen, the food, are institutionalized—"you can't bring it all in your suitcase!" I think back on Paula's birth experience. She had planned ahead—freezing the meal to be served after the birth, letting her mother-in-law know what kind of tea she preferred—had prepared her home for this event. She had her own things. She drank her tea from her own cup. This special cup was made by a friend who molded it especially for her. It was a clay cup with the iron particles showing through the glaze. It was round and smooth, nice to hold. During her labor, this cup, given with warm soothing tea, or with refreshing cool water, expressed the care and nourishment that Paula needed to be reminded of as she endured her trial. The cup tied her to her friends, and to the support that was needed to surround her during the pain. How different this cup is from the styrofoam cup often used to bring a woman nourishment during labor in the hospital.

Following One's Own Impulses

Many women talk of wanting to control the birth process. They want to be in control of their own experiences. In fact, the emphasis of many childbirth classes is to teach women how to use breathing patterns, controlled relaxation, or prepare written birth plans, in order to maintain as much control as possible. And it was control that the birthing room parents said they valued. Yet, one has to wonder what this focus on control is really about. Is it really control that is desired?

To be able to "go with" labor and its pain, one has to lose control to let the body do its work, to ride the wave of the pain. Perhaps in order to gain control one has to lose it. A strange possibility. Yet, if women know they have control of their environment, they may be more free to abandon inner control and follow the "out-of-control-ness" of their laboring body. In such a supportive environment women would be able to pick up "control" again when they choose (Morgan 1984). In such an environment the fear of losing control would not be an issue.

It may appear from this discussion that the home is the best place to birth a child; however, in many present situations, the home may not be a good place at all. What is important is that women need to feel comfortable enough (like they are when they are at home) so that their need to express their pain through change of position, having friends and family near, making noise, or receiving medication, is supported. The birthing room concept has the potential to provide such an environment—a place where women can truly be "at home" in the hospital, a place where she may follow her own impulses without the fear of losing control.

COMMUNITY SUPPORT DURING PAIN

Neumann (1955) and Briffault (1927) found that taboos initiated by women and imposed on themselves and men included the monthly "segregation" in the closed sacral precinct during their menstrual period. "Childbearing occurred in this same precinct, which was the natural, social, and psychological center of the female group, ruled over by the old, experienced women" (Neumann 1955: 290). In that earlier culture the knowledge of the effect of herbs and fruits was used to soothe the pain. Even today other women's knowledge and experience of childbirth pain helps the childbearing woman face her own pain.

> I thought of the millions, literally billions of women who have experienced this pain, and if they could experience it, then I can too. That made me feel strong—that all women go through this. (A4)

Jane, too, took strength in the fact that other women have gone through and continue to go through this experience. The knowledge that women share with other women has been lost in the replacement of midwives by doctors (primarily male) as birth attendants. This loss is being recognized. The challenge by women to regain control of the childbirth process is a recognition of the importance of sharing the bodily knowing of childbirth with other women, as a mother would.

> My friend told me several times that I did well. Part of me wants to reject this because of the feeling that I wasn't controlled, I was lazy, I didn't perform ideally the way I imagined I would. Yet, overwhelmingly, I want to believe her and I do believe her. After all, I DID IT! It was hard. It was long. I did rely on my instincts. I did rely on my friends. In a very real sense, we did it together. After my first child, I felt, and continue to feel, that I'd always have an affinity with other women, unnamed but real. (P2)
>
> If women don't have a husband who took the time to know as much as Mike did—if they don't have somebody with them who really knows what's going on—how really, really vulnerable and devastating an experience it could be. (K3)
>
> I can't begin to envision the nightmare and horror of carrying on (in the pain) without being in an atmosphere of caring and loving people. (P2)

Another woman said, "I did need help, I really needed help. It gets to the point that you need help for really simple sorts of things." Such support must be there without the asking.

Many woman choose the hospital as the place for birth because they have come to see themselves as safe in that environment. The experts and technology are there if needed. Women recognize their need for support. They need to know that they are doing well. They need support from partners and friends as well as the experts. Support may take the form of back rubs, direct suggestions, sips of cool water, a cup of warm tea, a soothing touch, the words of encouragement, the presence of a caring person, the quiet of the room, and an acknowledgment that what is happening is normal and expected. Women need to be reminded that the pain is there because pain is integral to the nature of birthing, not necessarily because something is wrong.

While there needs to be direct verbal and physical support, there also needs to be recognition and respect for the privacy of the pain. As Paula said, "I especially appreciated everyone's silence while I rested on my side— I knew people were with me—there was never a doubt in my mind" (P2). Yet in this inwardness there is an attentiveness to the deep significance of the momentous quality of the pain. This is important pain, "a sacred fire." One woman said, "I was annoyed when someone was making light conversation with my husband. I felt it was disturbing and irrelevant to what was happening to me" (L). Another said, "I couldn't talk, didn't want to. In fact, I wanted to be alone at this point" (H).

> It was an incredible sensation being totally into myself. I didn't have thoughts. I was really in tune with my body. I think it must be something in you that just happens. In meditation you can go so far but this was much, much different. In those last few hours there was no straying of the mind. I couldn't talk because I was on one plane and he was on another. Mine was an inward focus. (V)
>
> I was aware that the midwife looked at me intensely and I couldn't bear to respond—I think my reaction was part of being inward—to respond would have removed me somewhat from what I was feeling. (P2)

This deeply felt experience reaches to the core and, as Buytendijk (1961) said, "throws us back on ourselves." It demands women to muster up even more strength to survive, to live through it.

But not alone. "I look at Marie and I see the terror of childbirth in her eyes. I feel it. I remember it. I know it can be survived. I tell her so" (Harrison 1982: 105). In aiding the laboring woman, one must recognize her autonomy and the reality of pain and difficulty. One must encourage her to use her special capacities to deal with the pain as a creative action of nature and not as oppression (Kittay 1983: 124). For example, comments like "Perhaps you need a sedative," may lead to personal doubt and loss of confidence. Is it possible that the offer of medication to obliterate pain is sometimes accepted by a woman as it is the only support that is offered in the face of the overwhelming sensation of the pain? The offer of medication confirms the fear that, yes indeed, she will not be able to stand it. There is nothing else to do but suffer or be medicated. This is not to say that a woman does not need the help of medication—but the offer of medication (knowing its harmful potential for baby and mother) should not be the first or, indeed, the only support that is extended.

While recognizing the need for a supportive community during the painful birth experience, a woman may begin to grasp the reality of her aloneness. As she is surrounded by the deep sense of inwardness, she is compelled to acknowledge her independence, her selfhood, to be conscious of her own existence. "I feel great for the process to have happened through my body, proud of realizing such stamina, strength, and determination" (V). The woman learns about the strengths she has. She has climbed a mountain— reached a summit. She understands her own strengths and capabilities in a new way.

THE TIME OF PAIN

"And so it was, that, while they were there, the days were accomplished that she should be delivered" (Luke 2:6). It's time! Her time has come! The baby is coming! The pains tell the time. As the pains begin, women feel excitement. They also feel apprehension. This is what they've been waiting for. This is it! The pains are the knowing that the time has come. Yet, what is known? Women may know the stages of labor, know the procedures to expect, know some things to do, and yet ask, "How will I handle it? What will it *really* be like? Each time, we know more about what to expect and do, but the mystery of *this* time is still present. Each time is its own time.

Rhythm

"It is a different kind of pain—like muscle cramps or extremely bad gas— comes and goes—that is the reward—that it goes away" (J3). Further exploration of the etymology of the word "birth," shows that "to bear children" is tied to the root *bara* (Old Norse), meaning wave, billow, or bore. "Bore" is defined as "a high and often dangerous wave caused by the surge of a flood tide upstream in a narrowing estuary or by colliding tidal currents. "This wave imagery is closely associated with the idea of rhythm. . . . With each wave of the sea the tide gradually flows farther in, bringing nearer the time when her baby will be in her arms" (Kitzinger 1979b: 85). We can have with the pain wave of birthing a sense of being carried by the pain as we ride with it, by being caught by the pain and enduring it, or by being overwhelmed by the power of the pain that "throws us upon the beach only to pull us out again to sea." The contractions of birthing, like the colliding of the tidal currents, are most painful at the point in the process when the baby moves down the "narrow estuary" of the birth canal. Birth, as wave, tells us about the coming and going of the pain, the developing intensity, the climax, the release, and the moment of gathering resources for the next coming of the pain wave.

When women talk about the time of labor, they think of timing the contractions:

And then about 9:30 P.M. I was thinking about my pains and noticed that one was coming from the back. I began to think I was in labor. We started to time them, 7 minutes, 10 minutes, and then about 10:30 they went to about 4 minutes, lasting about 30 or 60 seconds. It wasn't hard for me. (C3)
When I first went into labor it was about midnight—about 5 minutes apart, these funny twinges. (S3)
On Monday night I felt twinges, menstrual cramps—then the next day they were 10 minutes apart and about 30 seconds long. (A4)
Taking out our little brown spiral notebook which I had bought two days earlier, small enough to fit in a shirt pocket, he wrote down the time and duration of the contraction. He had a digital watch and used the lap counter, as if he were running. (Israeloff 1982: 86)

The timing of the contractions gives helpful hints as to what is happening, for we know that as the pains get longer and stronger the farther into labor the woman has progressed. Yet even this timing can be overdone, with pages of records of contractions, for after a point, most women know themselves the nature of their contractions. The more women are assisted to recognize their own body rhythm, the more they may be able to flow with its pain in the process of birthing their children.

It Would Never End

"It was as if the pain was all there was. It would never end. There would be no result. I would live it forever (P2). During labor there is no sense of growth and change but the cessation of time. There is no intention, only the will to endure. "I only know that I have been lying in this pain, concentrating on staying above it, for a long time because the hands on the clock say so, or the sun on the wall has moved to the other side of the room" (Young 1984: 54).

THE BABY AND THE MOTHER

The Baby

And then I couldn't believe the sensation because—it was—as soon as I saw him, it was as if everything was gone and it gets very blurry. (S4)
I couldn't take my eyes off him. I cut the cord. That was really cutting the cord, really making the break from the baby. It's one relationship—

then he is born—that relationship dies and another relationship begins. (V)

Deliver, deliverance, the act of transferring to another. The pains are a literal expression of the narrow gateway leading to release in the expanse of life. The involvement changes from the self-as-world to baby-as-world. As the body releases the baby, the pain is released. The attention is turned to the new life, the new being.

> When Joanna was placed on my tummy, I almost felt as if I couldn't react . . . as if I was slowly emerging from a situation of being purely reactive to what was overwhelming me (the pain) to coming back to "me" in all senses (the intellectual, the person others know, the daily self). In a way I was numbed and had to slowly make my way back into the world. (P2) Something in me was released. I turned away from my somewhat egotistic involvement in my labor toward my child, since that moment my love has grown so that . . . it actually hurts sometimes. (Kitzinger 1977: 161)

The pain is released, with the possibility of a new and different pain tied to the incredible and awesome awareness of a separate being. The woman who becomes mother vastly increases her capacity for pain and vulnerability.

The Mother

"Being born into motherhood is the sharpest pain I've ever known" (Chesler 1979: 281). With the pain of childbirth women become mothers. Can pain be transformed into something usable, asked Rich (1976: 151), "something which takes us beyond the limits of our experience itself—into a further grasp of the essentials of life and the possibilities within us?" What is it that is learned?

> I think I have a right to feel good about myself. In a way, this birth is helping me to accept myself—both the limitations and the capabilities. Accepting myself is the other side of the coin of accepting the pain. I need to think further about it but have a sense that, for me, *this* has considerable significance. (P2)
> I would never have wanted it any other way. It gave me confidence and strength. I was able to deal with the pain, to confront and overcome. Now I know that I can deal with it—and that is useful in encountering other painful things. Of course, not all pain has a silver-lining—like the babe. (A6)

To have experienced birthing pain offers the possibilities of self-knowledge, knowledge of limitations and capabilites, knowledge of new life as mother, and of a woman's place in the mysterious cycle of human life: birth, death, and rebirth. As women give birth to children, they, in a sense, birth themselves. They become mothers, like their own mothers, and as their daughters will after them.

There is that sisterhood. There is a knowing that you, as a mother, have gone through what I've gone through. Men haven't gone through that— even though they participated as much as they could have. (A5)

Victoria said, "Rose was the only other mother there. I had something in common with her. I started to cry when she hugged me." (V)

Chapter 6

One for Another: The Transformative Sense of Responsibility

THE MEANING OF RESPONSIBILITY

To become a mother involves responsibility, responsibility for the birth and life of another person, the child. It can feel like an overwhelming responsibility—a terrifying one—especially when something goes wrong. An incident sticks in my mind from when my son was small. He was younger than four—sick with a cold or flu—his fever was rising. I felt his forehead, soothed his restlessness, wondered what to do. My hand moved to his pulse— a jolt went through me—his pulse was rapid and erratic, fitful, all over the place! What did this mean? Oh, No! Was something wrong with his heart? How did that happen? What can I do now?

We talk about taking responsibility for ourselves, and for the child, as Anna did during pregnancy, but when there is an actual child in your life, your child, a child entrusted to you (and even the child as stranger), who is not breathing properly, who has an erratic heartbeat, who is heard crying amidst the rubble of an earthquake, one is transformed by a sense of responsibility that subjects one to a certain terror that is not present in talk. Christine felt it early when she found herself bleeding, and Susan, too, when she thought her pregnancy might be tubal (the fertilized ovum implanted in the Fallopian tube which would mean surgery and the loss of her "baby"). And when Jena did not respond immediately at her birth, Bill had a sense of panic with the recognition that, "Oh, my gosh, is this what having a kid is like? Terror like this?"

We are shocked by our helplessness as we come face to face with the reality of illness, deformity, or death of the child we accepted in our life. "It took the wind right out of our sails," said the father of a two-year-old boy who needed chemotherapy treatment to live. "We want to take the pain and the treatment for him." Other parents say they would die that their child might live. What leads to a sense of responsibility that has such profound dimensions? Is this what having a child is like?

Thinking of responsibility in relation to becoming a mother, the following statement does not seem so strange, "Oh, yes we are finding baby furniture now, preparing, getting ready . . . and there is preparation for death too. Are they really so different" (Woodman 1985: 140)? As we prepare for a child in our life, we prepare to accept that something can go wrong. We are forced to imagine the death of our child. We are forced to face our own mortality. As we begin to acknowledge our own death, our thoughts come back to the child for whom we are responsible. Do I ever think of dying? Only in terms of who will mother my children. But then, how does one think of dying? One can only really think of living. Dying is too far away, or too close. "Who will mother my children?" A child needs a mother. In thoughts of death are we not reminded of life, of how we should live? In being responsive to our child and his or her life, are we not thrown into a renewed attention to how we should live? What has been a self-regulated, self-defined, and self-contained life is now suddenly broken by the experience of the Other, the child. And in taking responsibility for the child as Other, we are forced to be responsible also for ourselves. About a month before Keith's birth, Susan talked of her concern about Paul being away on a skiing trip which had never bothered her before. Now she says, "This child needs a father"(S2)! Or one can think of the father who stops drinking coffee to protect his heart, "I need to live at least until the boys are old enough to look after themselves." Even when Christine thinks of the possibility of the death of her baby, or her husband (given a choice), it is her son that should live (C7).

For a woman becoming a mother, this responsibility starts early. Even before Katherine knew for sure that she was pregnant she said, "I shouldn't be drinking now. It would be an inappropriate thing to do" (K1). In response to the baby they carry, women are subject to self-denial. Is this responsiveness not really a transformed experience of responsibility for the Other, the child? Can we get a clue from the origin of the word "responsibility"? "Responsible" comes from the Latin *respondēre*, "to promise in return." As we respond to the presence of the child, then, we promise to look after that child, to be trusted by the child, to care for the child, to return always. No longer are we acting only for ourselves—we are "one for the other" (Olson 1986). It is an awesome project.

A child needs a mother. By being responsive to a child in her life as Other, a woman becomes a mother. Yet, in that responsiveness there is a problem in living one's life solely for one's child. Recall Christine talking about women who seem to have lost themselves. "Everything is for their children or someone else and not for them" (C1). Here is the crunch, the dichotomy. How does a woman become responsible as a mother? How does a woman come to live as mother—for her child—and yet for herself? How does a woman act responsively toward the child in her life, and yet be true to herself and her own project of living? Does it mean that a woman gives her body completely over to the care of others during pregnancy? Does it mean that a woman's own experience of giving birth is secondary to the experience of birth for the child? Does it mean that a woman should stop her own projects and devote herself to the care of her child full-time? Does it mean that a woman should stop being in relation to other adults on a daily basis?

The situation of women in patriarchal societies complicates the matter further. Women are the "other"—like children, like blacks, like the aged, even like the poor. But here the notion of *other* is not that of the "real" Other, the child, which both women and men come to accept in parenthood. When writers like de Beauvoir, Daly, and O'Brien speak of women as "other," they remind us that women live in a world focused on the norm of the male body (not subject to the cyclical nature of menstruation), the male-dominated public decision-making bureaucracy (which venerates objectivity, management, control, and efficiency), and the male-dominated health care establishment (in terms of prestige and power).

For many women facing the responsibility of the child, the move to mother in the economic, political, and social sphere can be either empowering or disenfranchising—and in some sense, may be both. At the same time as a woman may feel blessed by a child in her life, by the very fact she is a mother, she may be even more oppressed. Poverty, lack of employment opportunities, lack of parenting support services such as flexible work hours, child care, or even financial assistance, make the endless tasks that are involved in caring for the young child very difficult. So for women, while they move toward a responsibility that transforms (in their responsiveness to the positive "other," the child), they are continually faced with the reality of their own "other"-ness (a negative reality) in our patriarchal culture. Therefore, in exploring the theme of responsibility, the focus becomes divided: responsibility for the baby, and responsibility for the woman. Should not both be considered? What is best for the baby cannot be overlooked, but what is good for the woman must also be kept in mind. Yet, in the effort to see the baby as central, there is the danger of the woman losing herself. As we realize responsibility to the child, as mother, the experience of self, as woman, becomes blurred.

TAKING RESPONSIBILITY

To have a healthy baby, the pregnant woman must be healthy. She is told by everyone—doctors, nurses, family, and friends—that she now must look after herself. As soon as she is pregnant, or even before, the woman is encouraged to eat right, avoid alcohol, tobacco, drugs, and even coffee. She is encouraged to get enough sleep, enough exercise, and enough fresh air. She is warned against micro-waves, computer monitors, X-rays, ultrasound, too much exercise, and even "You shouldn't lift things over your head" (B1). Women are becoming more conscious of the association between environmental and substance toxins, and fetal abnormalities. They are aware that their responsibility tends to come earlier and earlier, even before there may be any experience of pregnancy. Preconception information encourages this early responsiveness on the part of women.

So women look after themselves, in a way they did not before pregnancy, or the choice to have a child. When Christine found out that her blood pressure was fluctuating, she realized that she had to slow down.

> I'm more conscious of the pace, how I go through my day. If I am tired—well, I don't do the two other things I planned. I do what I have to do but I don't do the extra. I needed to be made aware of that—pay attention to my body. (C1)

Some women may find it easier to quit smoking when there is "someone else" to think about. Yet, some may not. They may become more responsive, and responsible, once they are convinced that there is a baby present. When they feel the movement, hear the heart beat, and see the kicks and rumbles across their stomachs, they begin to sense the reality of the baby. For some, ultrasound makes the baby's presence more real. "I had an ultrasound at eleven weeks. The baby was all there. Whole. It came real to me because of that. I didn't feel pregnant [but] it brought everything into focus" (C1).

Perhaps those women who do not stop smoking or drinking have not yet been transformed by that sense of responsibility for the child. This may seem like a simplistic notion, but it may be that women have not yet realized or believed that the child, as a separate being (but not independent), can truly be affected by their own actions. Is the "It cannot happen to me," another way of avoiding responsibility? The women in this study stopped drinking, watched their diet, and avoided "smoking environments" during pregnancy. They were doing this for their child, although Brenda talked about doing it for herself too. She said, "I figure that I have to look after this child so if it is healthy and happy it will be a lot easier" (B1).

But "taking care" may not be enough. The increasing number of technological investigations, such as amniocentesis and ultrasound, are constant reminders that in spite of their care of themselves women may bear a baby with congenital disease and handicaps, or that they themselves may develop high blood pressure, toxemia, or other diseases of pregnancy which could threaten their baby and themselves. Although Susan faithfully ate her "veggies," as she said, she was still afraid that her body would let her down, and her baby would not make it. Anna too, looked after herself with care, but worried about the possibility of a deformed child, "I don't know how I would deal with it—living with a child that has mental or physical problems on a day-to-day basis" (A1).

Susan had always had it in her mind to have a baby. In spite of the decision that now was the time, Susan did not conceive after trying for over two years. She and Paul applied to adopt a child. They decided to bring "any" child into the space they had opened for "their" child. Therefore, it came as a surprise for Susan when she became pregnant. She was cautious, however. She did not trust her body and dared not be too open to this child. "I have not bought any baby clothes, or that kind of stuff. I have been prepared for the worst that I sort of don't want to push it. It is too early, like it is going to be jinxed" (S1). She saw "the little heart beating," through ultrasound at eleven weeks and felt the baby move, but still held back. "The worst" might still happen. So Susan, at the same time as she wanted a child in her life, would not let herself really be at ease in accepting the reality of "this" child. It was not until the eighth month that the space for the baby in the house was ready. Now she could say, "Yeah, I've got the curtains done and I've got the quilt-cover done, and the crib is painted. You see if worse came to worse and I delivered the baby now, there's a pretty good chance that, you know, things could be okay. And so I feel a little more like going and looking for baby things" (S2). Although women have a sense of their own responsibility in creating a healthy baby, there is also the realization that there are things about having a baby that are beyond their control.

Getting Things Ready

As many women get closer to the time of birth, they begin to feel their responsibility to get things ready—the baby's clothes, the baby's room—and they also get ready for their own labor experience. They pack their bag. And in their bag they may have a Birth Plan that they have worked out with the doctor. They have chosen the person, usually the child's father or a close woman friend, to be with them. They are ready.

Yet when Anna talked of taking the responsibility for the birth, she described how she had sterilized the towels and sheets, how she had purchased the protective sheet for the bed, and even, early on, how she had found a place to live that would accommodate the home birth. She said, "It was almost a ritual to sterilize the towels and things. It was good to do that because to a certain extent you're overwhelmed by the responsibility. I don't think I would encounter that if all I did was to pack a bag and go to the door of the hospital. It is a different kind of preparation" (A2). The actual physical preparation (sterilizing the towels and purchasing the pads) helped Anna to prepare to take the responsibility for giving birth.

Anna was the only mother in this study who talked about the possibility of the death of her child during labor and delivery. It was central to her story. Of course, this was understandable since she had chosen to birth her child outside the bounds of "approved" practice. Thus she was open to all the "what if" questions that hospital care is presumed to deflect. Anna said, "I have thought of the potential of—let's say the baby doesn't make it. If it [the birth] is in the hospital everyone would say that the doctor tried his very best, but if that happened at home, we are going to be seen as irresponsible—as killers, or murderers" (A1). Then she said, "I think that for us a birth at home is less of a risk than the hospital. I think people do not want to believe that it is safer at home because they want to put the responsibility into the hands of the doctor and the hospital." Anna would say, then, that having the baby at home and getting things ready for the birth helped her to move to motherhood through accepting responsibility for herself and her child in a way that she could not if she had planned to go to hospital. Of course, she said that she would go to hospital if necessary, but would prefer to stay home.

The women were ready when the time came. The frequent trips to the bathroom, the difficulty in moving around easily, the need to eat small, more frequent meals, the finding a comfortable position for sleep, all made each woman ready.

> Now the baby has filled up the space, very tight—my stomach is lopsided sometimes—with head and foot sticking out. (C2)
> I'm feeling more discomfort. You know, up until Christmas it was easy. But since then, I've been feeling more and more sluggish and slow. I guess if you felt wonderful until the end you wouldn't care if you had the baby out or not. But, you know, whenever it is ready to come out, I'm ready. (S3)

But what does it mean to be ready? While Susan thinks it is time for the birth, that her body is ready, she also wonders about her readiness in another sense.

> Gee, am I ready for this? I am going to be 32, I'd better be ready. When are you going to be ready. I think as soon as we have the baby I'll feel like—I think it's like starting any new job, you know, I didn't feel like a teacher until I started doing it." (S3)

EMBODIED RESPONSIBILITY

Woman are made ready by experiencing the responsibility through their bodies. Many are aware of their pregnancy before they "know for sure" from a pregnancy test, or the doctor's examination. Christine was so sure that, in spite of the fact that the pregnancy test was negative, she said to her doctor, "Treat me as if I am because I am" (C1). Katherine, also, was sure, so she didn't need to purchase the pregnancy kit that contained two tests. One would do. Susan, on the other hand, had lost faith in her body, was fed up with her body not doing things right so she did not consider her very sore breasts—so uncomfortable that she had a hard time walking up and down stairs—as a possible sign of pregnancy. Women depend on the doctor's examination for confirmation. Yet, dependency on the pregnancy test, the doctor's examination, and other recent technological devices, such as ultrasound, may devalue their own body-knowledge.

During labor this attitude can be especially problematic. A pregnant woman feels the contractions of her uterus and the movements of the baby with an immediacy and certainty that no one else can share, but with increasing use of techniques and machines such as ultrasound and fetal monitoring, her experiential knowledge is reduced in value, replaced by what is seen as more reliable knowledge. As devalued knowledge it is easy for a woman to lose touch with or doubt her own experience, and to accept objective knowledge as more correct and therefore valuable.

Body as Beyond Control

Menstruation is a sign that reminds women, and society, that complete control of female bodies is not possible. Perhaps this is why it is viewed so negatively by a society which, above all else, venerates control (Martel and Peterat 1985). This desire to control is so entrenched that the "sign" of menstruation is denigrated in the effort to control it. In pregnancy, the woman shares her body with the growing child, an experience bound by fatigue, weight gain, nausea, flatulence, shortness of breath, vulnerability, and clumsiness that can be only partially controlled. In fact, these uncomfortable bodily experiences are a part of a healthy pregnant woman's life. Labor has been defined as stages in an effort to manage and predict, but each woman's labor has its own rhythm, pattern, and progression that left alone passes in its own time. The baby, too, with a rhythm all its own, demands that time move with its pace ("fetal time" as it is called by Rapp 1984: 314). The effort to control, for example, to control death, especially the death of a baby, creates dilemmas that now confront us, like the "right to die," which might be equally as important as to "live at all costs" (Colen 1986; McDermott 1986).

Humility, the virtue needed to take on a world beyond our control, "emerges from maternal practices and accepts not only the reality of damage and death, but also the actuality of the independent and uncontrollable life of nature" (Ruddick 1983: 217). Humility, when confused with self-efface-ment (humility's degenerative form), is a negative image that mothers and society abhor. Nevertheless, true humility, developed in face of the circum-stances of life's uncontrollable situations, is a characteristic to be treasured. Faith in women's bodies gives power, not power "over" but power to "go with," to move within the forces of body knowledge. Such faith gives women the confidence needed to take charge of their own environments which allows for freedom to live autonomously, to be self-reliant, and to make individual choices in line with their own sense of values (Kitzinger 1975). Women who mother are transformed by the recognition that complete control of life, as the control of death, is an illusion (Greer 1985: 18).

Obstetrical science does not easily place itself in a humble relationship to the reality of the puzzle of life (which includes death), and those aspects that are out of human control (Young 1987). In the effort to control and manage life (and death) there is the potential for usurping the need of women to develop their own sense of responsibility that giving birth entails. Brenda's husband's wish for a cesarean birth gives a clue to the problem that is faced by women. Brenda said, "Now he wants me to have a cesarean so he could watch them take it out from the other side. He says it is more humane, like he didn't like to have the woman suffer" (B2). While it is important to control suffering, there is also a need to consider that the challenge faced by women in childbirth, in the experience of labor, may have value that comes with accepting responsibility.

Cesarean Births

Close to one out of every five births in Canada and the United States now occurs by cesarean section (Elkins 1983: 2; Cohen and Estner 1983: 9; Brack-bill et al. 1984: 23). There are situations in which the cesarean birth is necessary to save the life of the baby or woman, such as maternal pelvic contraction, prolapse of the cord, and hemorrhagic conditions (Cohen and Estner 1983). There are other situations in which cesarean sections are not so easily justifiable, such as dystocia, prior cesarean delivery, and breech presentation (Young 1987). With the declining birth rate, and the fact that many women wait longer before having a baby, the perfect baby is sought as never before. Some women and doctors expect that the cesarean birth increases the probability of having the "perfect" baby, and almost always the cesarean section is done on behalf of the child (Brackbill et al. 1984: 23–25). "When it's an older woman and there is a chance that this is the only child she will have, you want to make sure it is alive and well. So I call a halt to the risk taking much earlier through surgical intervention," said one doctor (Fabe and Wikler 1979: 287). This means that the "risk-taking" of the vaginal birth is being replaced by the "risk taking" of surgical birth—an interesting notion. The "out-of-control-ness" of women's bodies is devalued in search of perfection and control. Obstetrical science and technology are thought to be more reliable and predictable than the vaginal process of giving birth. Here, control of the natural process is dominant. No thought is given to the woman's need to birth the child through her body. No thought is given to the process of birth as a valuable, and perhaps essential, part of a woman's transformation to mother. No thought is given to the idea that knowledge of childbirth is valuable knowledge for society as a whole. Raising concerns about cesarean births does not disregard the fact that some babies or mothers may need this intervention. Rather, the concern is raised to question the notion that surgical intervention may be thought of as a better way to birth.

Katherine, like other cesarean-birth mothers described in Cohen and Estner (1983), spoke of the disappointment and guilt she had about her cesarean delivery. Katherine said to Brett, her baby, many times, "I'm sorry, kid, that it happened like that" (K4). Katherine talked of her sadness and the real sense of the inadequacy in her body, that her "body let her down." Another woman may say, "What did I do wrong?" Perhaps these uncomfortable feelings have to do with the lack of "bonding-time" (especially with general anesthesia), or of being denied the opportunity to see and hear the baby right away. Or perhaps the disappointment comes from missing the feeling of the baby moving out of the woman's own body. In contrast to these voices, Jane said that her acceptance of responsibility was partly due to the birth itself, "I suppose part of it is working towards having the baby—doing all that hard work—and then seeing this baby come out of your own body in birth. It was seeing her" (J3). The actual birthing experience, the labor itself, may be important to women. Maybe it is seeing the "whole picture" as Katherine said (K3). The woman wants to find out what really happened. She wants to see what the obstetrician wrote on her chart. She wants to see what her baby was like at birth (that is, the Apgar score). She wants, in a sense, to re-live the birth. The birth process, her labor, is important for her own understanding of herself as mother.

The desire to control nature is not new. To control nature, to try to improve on women's ability to deliver babies vaginally, is the expected result of the never-ending search to control life. Think back on an earlier example in this book regarding the practice of separating infants and mothers at birth. Although some women wanted babies with them, it was not until there was scientific "proof" of the value of those initial hours that the "natural" was supported by the "scientific" so that practices changed. At the present time, a woman like Brenda who is not able, for whatever reason, to look at or reach for her baby at birth, is observed by the staff as a concern to be "noted on the chart." Prior to the scientific research on bonding, Brenda's reaction would have not been thought so significant. Will scientific studies be needed to convince the obstetrical surgeons that the vaginal birth is a better way for living as humans for both babies *and* mothers? In spite of scientific medicine's impact on mortality rates and heroic life-saving practices, the significance of the vaginal birth for women needs to be reconsidered. In fact, it is precisely because the mortality rates have decreased that attention can be paid to the practices in childbirth in terms of what is right and good for our humanity, and what is right and good for women in their project of giving birth and becoming mothers.

In the effort to control nature for the perfect baby, what may be bypassed is the quality of life (the whole picture). The whole picture includes the child and the mother. Birth is not just for the child, or for the mother. It is a relational, a community activity. The mother's realization and acknowledgment of the strength and power of her reproductive body is realized in her ability to birth her own child. What may be lost in bypassing this event is the experience that is a necessary part of the reproductive cycle. Pregnancy and birth is likened to the progression and intensity of sexual pleasure in intercourse. What happens when women miss the orgasm, the release, that leads to satisfaction and contentment? What happens to women like Katherine who grieve because their bodies let them down? How do they work through their sadness so that they need not feel guilty about a process that was out of their control? That embodied experience of "giving" birth that enables women to learn to take the responsibility for the child may be missed in cesarean deliveries.

THE SPACE OF RESPONSIBILITY

Today much discussion about childbirth focuses on the place of birth. Most women and medical personnel agree that the hospital is the preferred location, primarily because of the proximity to life-saving expertise and machines. Women, generally, feel they are taking responsible action by following this trend. They do not wish to take a chance. Yet, there some women who are beginning to realize that the hospital environment may not be the most favorable place for this intimate event to take place. Christine and Brenda delivered in the traditional labor and delivery room system, while Jane and Susan delivered in a birthing room. Both Anna and Katherine chose to deliver their babies at home. Anna and Katherine felt that a home birth offered the opportunity for them to act on their own good judgment rather than under the authority of others, such as the doctor and hospital staff. The issue is not the question of safety: both women felt they were making choices based on the literature that states that with a normal birth, the home is as safe, or even safer, than a hospital (Mehl, Peterson, Whitt, and Hawes 1977; Hoff and Schneiderman 1985).

All the women spoke of childbirth as a normal, natural event. Up until the time of the birth all took responsibility for themselves—they watched their nutrition, they exercised, they went for their regular checkups, and they took prenatal classes. Yet, like most women, Brenda, Christine, Jane, and Susan, chose a place of birth in which they would be safe in the hands of others. Of course, it may be that in our present health care environment, without adequate medical support in the home, the hospital is the most appropriate choice. What does choosing a place of birth have to do with responsibility? Katherine hints at this question as she describes her move from home to hospital during labor:

> When I went into hospital things really changed for me in the sense that all of a sudden there were a lot of things done to me. I was a patient. It was a real change—a turning point. From then on things were really out of my hands. (K3)

"Things were out of her hands"—she was no longer in control. Did this mean she was no longer responsible?

Hospital Space: *"They did a lot to me"*

When I visited Brenda in the hospital the day after the birth, I was reminded of the fact that, although I was visiting her, both of us were visitors in the hospital. Brenda sat on "her" bed in a room with two or three other women. Suzie, her new baby daughter, was sleeping in a plastic bassinet at her side. Brenda felt well and talked about going home. She did not like the hospital—the bed, the place, the noise, the babies crying, and the things that kept them busy. She wondered about her husband, how he was and what he was doing. She was not "at home" in the hospital. It is a foreign space, someone else is in charge. In such an environment it becomes easily possible for "them" to do things to "you."

The rituals that occur in the hospital environment demonstrate how responsibility shifts from personal autonomy of the woman to authority and responsibility centered in the hospital staff and hospital routine (Kelpin and Martel 1984).[1] Etymologically, "hospital" is a doublet of "hotel" and the words presuppose that someone enters into a "hospitable" place, as a guest or a hostess. The hospital, as we know it, is the place where sick people enter in order to be restored to health or to die. Christine, the birth-giving, healthy, pregnant woman also entered the hospital.

> You know what struck me [she talks hesitantly] when you go through admitting, they are, uh, your name, number—("Don't you know I'm in labor!) It was so routine to them. The admitting was quite long, and I was getting quite uncomfortable, and I needed to lie down or something—and them asking for my social insurance number. I had forgotten it, and

now 'what do I do?' I just remember thinking that this must be very boring for them, this routine business. (C3)

Christine speaks of "routine business," of "numbers," and of the "boredom" of admitting staff. The exciting reality of labor for the woman, and the formal and routine reception of entering the hospital, were at odds. A wheelchair was brought down from the ward for Christine. "Did they think I needed a wheelchair?" she thought. Although not used, the presence of the wheelchair was a symbol of incapacity and a reminder that she was in a place for the weak, sick, and needy.

Next, Christine was taken "up to the ward." The word "ward" comes from the Anglo-Saxon *weardian*, meaning "to fend off, to keep from hitting, to turn aside anything mischievous that approaches." To be taken "up to the ward" literally means to be brought under guard in confinement or custody, to be brought up to protection. The ward is the perfect place to depend on others. She said:

Then things happened really fast, they did a lot to me. I can't tell you a lot of the things that happened between arrival and getting into bed. It's vague—I was really intent on lying down. I wanted to get into bed and to get relaxed. (C3)

Activity was all around her but she just wanted to relax. Christine's words display the gap between what she wanted to experience, that is, the relaxing of her body, and what was seen as necessary for her admission to the hospital. Her concentration was focused inward while the admission procedures forced her attention outward.

Her world on the ward becomes the world of the "they." They are the anonymous people, nurses whose names and faces she could not remember. They were introduced to her but she could not remember who they were. As her attention was turned inward, the people around her remained faceless and her surroundings remained vague. "It was a quiet room," said Christine, "I thought that was fine. It was fine for me to be by myself with my husband, or with them. I can remember getting the gown on. There were several nurses involved" (C3). Attired according to the status of a patient, Christine entered further into the world of medicine (of passivity and obedience). Her gratefulness at being in a quiet room alone with her husband shows Christine's underlying desire for autonomy or independence in an environment which would support her need for relaxation and inward attention.

The statement "they did a lot to me" shows a passivity suitable to patienthood on the ward. Like Katherine, Christine was becoming a "patient," from the Latin *pati*, "to suffer" as one who patiently waits upon the initiative of others who know what needs to be done. From the healthy condition of a life giver, she is transformed into the recipient of care within the enclosure and procedures of the hospital ward. Becoming a patient meant that she had lost her autonomy as an independent healthy person and gained dependence upon the medical community. What does this move to patienthood do to her own sense of responsibility?

Does the use of a birthing room change this gradual assimilation into the hospital environment and the "patienthood" that Christine and Katherine experienced? Susan and Jane used the birthing room. Both found it pleasant. Of course, so did Christine, for that matter. But here the attempt is to understand how women are transformed by the responsibility that becoming a mother entails, and how the environment for the birthing supports or hinders that process.

The staff at the hospital where Susan birthed left her and her husband, Paul, alone much of the time during labor, after checking the fetal heart with the stethoscope. Susan's main concern during labor was that she did not make too much noise. She wanted to fit in without a fuss. The staff were supportive and gave her ice water for her dry mouth, *Demerol* for her pain (which did not relieve the pain but made her dozy and distant from it), and helped her find comfortable positions for labor. The fetal monitor was not used. In the end, Susan needed the help of forceps to bring the baby's head over the lip of the cervix which would not retract. The staff were there to help Susan and seemed to consider her wishes (for example, delaying the rupture of the membranes), and Susan was grateful for the care they gave her. The five days she spent in the hospital went quickly. It was a busy time. "By the time you fit yourself around the hospital's schedule—breakfast at a certain time, and then exercises, and then the baby is brought in to be bathed and fed—there is not much time left" (S4).

Jane arrived at the hospital about two hours before Lisa's birth and was pleased that the birthing room became available to her. "It was great," she said, "It was carpeted and there was music playing, with a little television beside the bed, and a telephone near" (J3). She was put on the fetal monitor right away, and once her membranes had been ruptured by the resident doctor, the external apparatus was replaced with internal electrodes. Jane thought the membranes were ruptured because they were so busy they needed the room and "didn't want me to take any more time than I had to." The nurses and doctors were helpful, giving directions to guide the birth.

> All of a sudden, in the middle of a contraction, I had to push. They said, "Don't push, don't push." I could breathe through those all right. My doctor was still not there, so the resident came back in and scrubbed, and got all dressed up, and kept saying, "Don't push, don't push." Then my doctor arrived and I was told to, "Breathe, breathe," until he was ready. So by the time I was allowed to push, I was really ready to push. Jim was really my saving grace, as he kept saying, "Don't push, breathe." He kept me on track. Even then, when I got pushing, they wanted me to stop so they could do an episiotomy. That was really tough. When she came out I was really amazed, she was so tiny yet she looked so big. The

head looks incredible. It was just more awe inspiring than anything. The doctor held her up, before they cut the cord, and said, "Look, don't touch, but look at her." And we looked at her. (J3)

Jim was Jane's saving grace—keeping her on track according to the directions and wishes of the doctors and nursing staff. Jane was only "allowed" to push when they were ready. Most of her labor was spent at home where it had progressed normally as she followed the rhythm of her laboring body in a supportive environment of her husband and parents. When she went to the hospital and moved toward birth (in the birthing room), she was told what to do so that the staff and their procedures could be accommodated—the waiting for the doctor, the scrubbing, the dressing, the episiotomy. Now she needed to be "kept on track," to look but not touch, and to be "saved" by others. When we think of Brenda, of Christine, of Susan, and of Jane, we remember that they all accommodated themselves to fit in to others expectations. Has the birthing room really enabled women to gain access to the life-saving capabilities of medical science without depriving them of their own life-giving prerogatives? In whose hands is birth?

Home Space: "We did it ourselves"

When I visited Anna the day after the birth of Jena, another situation was evident. Anna and Jena, along with Anna's sister Carol and her two-year-old daughter, Nicky, were together in their living room. Nicky held the baby. Anna served me coffee. A short time later Bill arrived with a big box of diapers. They were at home. I was the guest.

By virtue of it being their home, their space, they were in control. By being in control of their space, they were able to allow the birth process to proceed in its own time. Anna felt she was in control most of the time during her labor (although she nearly "lost it" in transition). Yet during the labor itself one really expects to lose control—the contractions of the uterus, the pain, the intensity take over, take charge—and by going with it, in a sense by losing control, one gains control.

> I was in my body. . . . I was somewhere on the ceiling, out of reach, out of hearing. My thoughts were in one place, my body in another. (Chesler 1979: 255)

"The midwives were incredible," said Bill, "they were so unobtrusive. They didn't do a lot during labor, they were so patient. It was wonderful to have them here—to check the fetal heart—but because we were managing, they stayed in the background" (A4). Bill goes on to say, "We did it ourselves," which is what, I think, women want when they say they want control. They want to do it themselves, they want to be self-reliant without losing the support of others. Bill's remark differs substantially from the misguided sense of responsibility exemplified in the doctor's comment to Christine after her birth, "I don't want you to do that to me again" (C3). Although Christine had maintained control of herself to the best of her ability, she was held responsible for the difficult labor (after being subtly subdued into patienthood and thus denied personal autonomy).

In the hospital it is easy for the doctors, the nurses, and others to take responsibility; it is their space. At home, although the midwives were there, the responsibility falls on the mother (parents); it is their space. No matter how the hospital rooms are "dolled up" (Anna's term) with the cozy quilt, the rocking chair, and the telephone, the home-like hospital is still a strange place, a foreign space—"might as well have the green walls and the harsh lights," said Anna (A6). A foreign space, by the very fact that it is not home, creates a problem of control, of "whose hands it is in." Yet again, perhaps it is not control at all that is desired, rather self-reliance—the difference is a tricky one. Even in the birthing room there is a need for staff to relinquish control so that a woman can be free to follow the intuitive knowledge embodied in her birthing body, to "go with" rather than to "manage" the birthing process. "For a woman to attain autonomy she need not renounce her biological capacities, but gain control over them" (Kittay 1984: 133). In gaining control she has the opportunity to relinquish her control to the autonomy of her own birth-giving body and its process.

Hospital environments can be made to be "home" away from home, not only with changed decor, but with a philosophy that puts women at the center. An excerpt from a letter, from a woman who birthed her child in Pithiviers Hospital in France, illustrates a supportive hospital environment where a woman can truly "give" birth.

> I am breathing like a toad: through the top of my throat. Dr. Odent comes in. The waters break. The midwife gently suggests I adopt a semi-squatting position, supported by Eddie. At first I am not too sure, but it does help. As each contraction overwhelms me, I am still moaning very loud, but just for the length of the contraction. Everyone else is calm, quiet, and supportive. Dr. Odent gives me lumps of sugar, for energy, and water (I drink about two pints in all). Suddenly I can feel the head coming down. I am glad because I am looking forward to sleeping, baby or no baby. While standing between contractions, I rock on my feet very gently. The head is visible. Eddie is supporting me. One push and I feel our baby coming out. The midwife catches her; I think she helped turn her slightly. My memory of that second is hazy with excitement. Eddie lowers me and they put the baby in my arms. I am stunned; not a word is spoken. The baby cries a bit and starts looking for the nipple. All is so peaceful and so intense. The midwife and Dr. Odent are in a corner, available, yet making themselves totally unobtrusive. The moment belongs to the three of us. (Odent 1984a: 56–57)

It is the woman who gives birth, within the arms of a caring partner, and with the assistance and support of knowledgeable people. Nothing has been taken away from her own process, and as she births the child she can begin to respond to that child, nourishing the child by offering the breast, and moving toward the responsibility of mothering.

RESPONSIBLE RELATIONSHIPS

Choosing a Doctor

One of the first things a woman does when she finds herself pregnant is to "choose a doctor," the care giver. The consumer process of "shopping around" for someone who will support a woman's needs, desires, and priorities is now encouraged by childbirth educators and consumer advocates. "The choice of care giver and a place of birth determine, to a great extent, the kind of birth experience you will have" (Simkin et al. 1984: 5).

Some doctors, according to Anna, want to take credit for the birth (A1). She and Bill, her husband, felt that their choice of doctor and midwife helped them to take their own responsibility for the pregnancy, birth, and the child. Recall Anna's comment about the chance of the death of their child—they would be seen "as irresponsible, as killers, and murderers" (A1). Pretty strong words. They would be responsible. It was different for Brenda. She said, "Whatever will be, will be" (B2). Everything was left to her doctor's discretion.

Susan was so concerned about the shared medical practice, with the possibility that a doctor she did not know would be present at the birth, that she decided to change doctors. Some of her nurse friends had warned her about doctors who "did episiotomies down to one's kneecaps." But Susan felt unsure of herself. Was it the pregnancy that made her feel so helpless? She thought, "How am I going to tell this man?" when she usually felt that one should stand up to the doctor. "I was more paranoid than I was before," and was grateful when the doctor, himself, suggested the referral (S1).

For many years pregnant women have been used to experiencing the effect of the attitude that the obstetrician should take over the guardianship of the woman for twelve months—"supervising food intake, regulation of activities, answering questions, clarifying puzzlements, and advising on handling the baby and generally charting her activities" (quoted in Seiden 1978: 92). Many women are not willing to accept such patronizing anymore but sometimes find it hard to achieve a healthy balance of cooperation with those to whom they go for care.

Take, for example, Christine's discussion with her doctor about the use of the fetal monitor during labor. Christine expressed surprise when she found out that at least one-third of the women in the hospital of her choice had the monitor during labor (C2). In discussing it with her doctor she felt that she had little choice but to accept what he wished to do, although either using or not using the monitor had problems according to the doctor's comments. Her doctor had said:

> The obstetricians, or whoever delivers, have lost their skill in being able to listen to the heartbeat, and to know what is going on—because it is so hard to hear externally. The heartbeat will go up and down, and race around, and some doctors panic when they hear it just externally and do a section needlessly. The advantage of the monitor is that you can then read the tape, and know. The same problem exists when you don't know how to read the fetal monitor, because you may then panic, (and those are the words he used) and jump in and do a section before you need to. (C4)

After this bit of ambivalence, the doctor said, "But if you don't want to be monitored I won't, but I would prefer it." (C4) Did Christine really have a choice?

"I Don't Want a Daughter"

There was often talk about the sex of the baby. Some of the women played around with the "needle" test—where a needle is hung on a string over the woman's belly and its movement (back and forth, or in circles) is said to indicate the sex of the baby. Some say this test may be just as accurate as guessing the sex by the rate of the fetal heart! Will the baby be a boy or a girl? Of course, it does not really matter. But does it? "We would be happy with either," said Brenda (B2). Yet at the same time she also said she would prefer a boy, primarily because she expected that her husband would treat a daughter differently from a son—like never letting her out of his sight, or questioning her about everything she did. Was she saying that she didn't want her girl to be treated as she was, having even simple decisions made for her?

Women realize that there is a responsibility to society to raise an acceptable child (Ruddick 1983). What kind of girl or boy is acceptable to present society? Christine, pregnant with her second child, said that this time:

> We would really like a baby girl. Yet I kind of think, you know what . . . [speaking very quietly], I kind of think I don't know if I want a girl, just because I don't know if I want her to face this world as a woman. I still think that men have an easier time. . . . I would want my little girl to just go for it, like I think I have—and then I get quite concerned about the kinds of things she is going to have to go through or over—get over— to be a person in this world. I have ambivalent feelings about it. It would be fine but. . . . (C7)

Christine thinks it would be easier to raise a boy, because you could be direct and tell him what the world is like. With a girl there would be more of a dilemma. "My little girl would learn from me—but I'd have to tell her, 'we do *this* here but in the real world *that* will happen'—I wonder if I could prepare my girl child for the world as well as I could my boy child" (C7).

Although Brenda did not speak about her concern in terms of woman's position in society, her statement is even stronger in terms of the lived reality of a woman's life. She knows that a girl would be treated differently from a boy, and she does not want that for her child. During our final conversation, I asked Brenda how she felt about this issue now. She said, "Now Tom says Suzie is going to be a nun, because he remembers how wild he was, and doesn't want his girl to get that kind of treatment" (B5).

The actual desire for sons over daughters seems hardly a problem in our society. Most parents say, "it doesn't matter, as long as the baby is healthy." Yet they want a balanced family, and after one or two daughters may wish for at least one son. The technology is available to create gender imbalances through the deliberate choice of the sex of the child. Technology (particularly amniocentesis) brings "the age-old patriarchal 'dream' of selecting children's sex very close to fulfillment" (Hoskins and Holmes 1984: 249)—in fact, it is no longer just a dream (Rothman 1987). It happens! Recognition of the value of women, of girl children, and their contribution to society must occur in the public arena if the hesitations that Christine and Brenda speak about are to be avoided. In a community that treasures girls and boys for their unique contributions, parents would not choose a boy over a girl or a girl over a boy, but would welcome every child, and help each of them grow to become an acceptable and valued member of that community.

Chapter 7

Living with a Child: The Transformative Experience of Having a Child on One's Mind

THE MEANING OF SELF IN "ONE FOR ANOTHER"

Ariel: Wherever I am, you're there too, hovering around my shoulders, I'm never alone. Not even when I'm lonely, and quite alone; in my study, or in another city. (Chesler 1979: 190)

Before Brett's birth, Katherine talked self-assuredly about her plans for her birth and her child. She thought out her life carefully, it seemed, like finding work that would support her while she raised a child. She was independent, a woman who did things her own way. She had strong opinions of how she would like to give birth based on research, reading, and talking with others. In fact, it was ten years earlier that Katherine first started thinking about a home birth after reading *Immaculate Deception* by Suzanne Arms (1975). She was delighted to find out there were practicing midwives in her own locality who could make the birth at home a possibility. But in living with Brett, through the cesarean birth and the first few weeks, Katherine began to doubt herself. Before the birth she had thought that a cesarean birth would not necessarily be a problem in the establishment of a good relationship with the baby "because the relationship starts in pregnancy." She said, "It may be that a cesarean section is a kind of interruption in that relationship, but I think you can establish as good, if not better, relationship with your child afterwards" (K2). Yet she seemed not so sure after. "As I say I've apologized to her I don't know how many times—'I'm sorry kid, that it happened like that' " (K4). She was saddened by the experience, she felt her body had let her down. Katherine elaborated:

> Motherhood is a guilt trip. You feel guilty about a whole bunch of things— you are responsible for so many things and it is impossible to be one hundred percent on top of them all. You think, 'that's what my job is now, you've got to do all those things.' It makes me feel guilty. (K4)

The baby crying, not sleeping, being gassy, being hurt by a pin, dressed the wrong way, as well as the cesarean birth triggered these uncomfortable guilt feelings. "What am I doing that's causing this to be like this? I shouldn't have done that—maybe it was the pizza" (K4).

It seems that Katherine is not unusual. Many women experience the same thing. Chicago noted that although things like a miscarriage, placenta abruptio, or a deformed child, may actually be out of women's control, many women said, "I felt it was somehow my fault" (1985: 76). To have a child on one's mind seems to put oneself in question, which can involve change, an inner change, in a woman's understanding of herself. "She [daughter] has forced me to confront dark places in my own soul—my desire to possess, to own; selfishness, or egocentricity; real doubts about the purity of my past loves, past actions" (Dowrick and Grundberg 1980: 79).

"Guilt" is the fact of being responsible for wrongdoing. What is it that mothers feel they are doing wrong? It is easy to understand that with the responsibility for "doing," that is caring for the child, that one might feel that the doing is wrong when the child cries, will not sleep, or seems in pain. It is the caring for the vulnerable, the helpless, the dependent, the crying infant that causes mothers to feel the guilt, even if what is happening is not in their immediate control. "That first week was certainly a time of feeling, 'Is this right, is that right, is he alright, am I alright?' (C4). Care of the dependent and needful Other results in the self-questioning that new mothers feel. Katherine said, "I've got Brett on my mind all the time. It's ongoing. It's fragmented my thinking" (K3).

> Ariel is a great teacher. Not only does he force me to *see* my limitations; he has me—kicking and screaming—accepting them. *More:* For the first time in my life, I'm learning about love . . . about what it takes to nourish, maintain human life. (Chesler 1979: 191)

The child is beyond our understanding because the child is beyond us (Smith 1984). The child is our own flesh and blood, yet the Other.

What has happened? We have lost control of ourselves. Our child issues from a deliberate act, but his [her] presence represents something beyond deliberation. For now there is more to life than what we know, it is mysterious. The child comes as a stranger, but a stranger that we ourselves have created. What makes a child so strange is that he [she] is so familiar. After all we made him [her]. He [she] is our flesh and blood. That is why his [her] otherness is so incomprehensible. The aim to understand the child more completely, to contain him [her], to control him [her] misses the point. (Smith 1984: 292, brackets added)

The focus turns to the child. Henceforth the woman's attention is divided.

THE GIVING BODY

"I guess I started to feel motherly when she responded to something I did— if I talked to her, she seemed to quiet—seemed to know I was there and able to comfort her" (K3). Jane thought that the feeling of being a mother came through the daily tasks of feeding and caring for the child. When my own child was about five months old I took him to the Health Clinic for immunization and a check-up. He was a healthy child, chubby and active. As the nurse weighed him and realized that he was still being nursed without the introduction of many other foods, she said to me, "Well, you are quite a cow, aren't you!" I was furious! I did not know that my anger was a reaction to the importance for me of my nourishing and life-giving abilities. In using the metaphor of a cow, the nurse probably did not know that the "Goddess as cow, ruling over the food-giving herd," is one of the earliest historical objects of worship (Neumann 1955: 123; Corea 1985: 60–61).

Nourishment

The ability of women to nourish is something to be cherished. It is important to the child and to the mother—it ties mother to her child in necessary ways.

> To nourish and protect, to keep warm and hold fast—these are the functions in which the elementary character of the feminine operates in relation to the child, and here again this relation is the basis of the woman's own transformation. . . . After childbirth the woman's third blood mystery occurs: the transformation of blood into milk. (Neumann 1955: 32)

The symbols that belong to the vessel character of the belly during pregnancy are enclosed forms (such as jar, kettle, or oven), whereas the symbols that belong to the vessel character of the breast are open in character (bowl, goblet, cup, and the Grail). These symbols accentuate the giving, protecting, warming aspect of the Feminine archetype of nourishment (Neumann 1955: 46–47).

> Body-vessel and mother-child situation—the positive elementary character of the Feminine—spring from the most intimate personal experience, from an experience that is eternally human; and even when it is projected into the ends of heaven and earth, it preserves its closeness to the central personal phenomenon of feminine life. (Neumann, p. 147)

How then does this nourishing aspect of the mother-child bond transform the woman? Is it this aspect that connects a woman to her child in such a way that from thereafter the "child is always on one's mind?"

Katherine talked about how she rushed home from shopping with thoughts of the child. "I felt it (in my breasts) if I was even just thinking about her. I would start to feel really full and kind of anxious to get home. I'd sometimes just forego doing something that I thought I would do, just to get home" (K4). Jane, too, remarked on the time it takes to really see the child as an independent person. "I left Lisa with Jim and I phoned when I got there fifteen minutes later and then rushed home. The ties are incredible. The umbilical cord is not really cut for the first while. Now I can go out and not worry about her as much—I don't need her in my sight so much" (J4). While the primary interest of mothers, early on, is the preservation and nourishment of this new life, it is not long before other interests, such as fostering the child's growth, and shaping an acceptable child also become important (Ruddick 1983: 219–23). These interests demand change on the part of the woman which involves moving away from the child.

Love

There is danger in trivializing mother love which negates it, puts it down, makes it something private, which may not be valued in the public world. From "a child only a mother could love," to the once-a-year accolades of Mother's Day, the love of the mother gets taken for granted. In its taken-for-granted-ness it becomes "naturally" a woman's duty and domain (Ehrensaft, in Trebilcot 1983). What is this special love, this love that mothers feel? How does it come about? How does this love affect the woman herself and her understanding of herself as mother?

> The love of children is not only the most intense of attachments, but it is also a detachment, a giving up, a letting grow. To love a child without seizing or using it, to see the child's reality with the patient, loving eye of attention—such loving and attending might well describe the separation of mother and child from the mother's point of view. (Ruddick 1983: 224)

Weaning, according to the dictionary, means the substitution of other than mother's milk for nourishment, but weaning also starts in other ways. It is being comfortable with someone else holding and soothing your baby, letting someone look after the child while you go out to dinner, or feeling comfortable with the child staying overnight with grandparents. Jane's admittance that she does not need Lisa in her sight so much may be an aspect of weaning—or when Anna responds to people who remark on Jena's beauty by saying, "Yes, she is, isn't she?," rather than, "Thank you." "After all," said Anna, "Jena is her own person, and should get the credit for being beautiful" (A6).

Christine talked of valuing David's own needs and working around his sleep patterns or eating patterns, or even just allowing him to be fussy if that is what he needed to do.

> When he cries, he gets terribly upset and that is hard, it is hard for me to hold him when he is doing that. I try to just hold and comfort him. . . . You just have to let him cry—as long as he is not choking or in danger— I just try to be here and let it happen. It is not easy. (C4)

In a legend of the Grail it is said that a king, paralyzed by a painful injury, offered the Grail to the first person who asked him, as the guardian of the Grail, "What are you going through?" The love of Other is that kind of love (Weil, as quoted in Ruddick 1983: 224), an attention and respect to what the child is "going through." This nurturing, thoughtful love is expressed by letting Jena feed on demand and acknowledging the child's own patterns of sleep. Within this love Anna is respecting the individuality of her child and the child's separateness from herself as the mother.

Yet in the weaning from the breast and the recognition of the separateness of the child, there is still the realization that the mother's body and her attentive love, hold an ongoing and lasting aspect of support for the child. Twelve years old, still a child and yet rapidly moving into the possibility of manhood, my son asked if he could sit in my lap. As his growing body covered my lap and my vision, he wondered how he was as a child in my lap. We laughed and tried different positions to capture again what it was like. He said "You know, this is my home!"[1] A mother's body gives the child the sense of home. The very fact that the woman's body carried and nourished the child ties a mother to her sons and daughters in a unique and intimate way. It does not mean, however, that women are alone in their giving of attentive love. It may be "naturally" theirs—but it may not be "only" theirs.

THE MOTHER CHILD BOND

The women talked of their first encounters with their children. Anna said: "Later on in the day she was born, I came in here and put some music on— and just kind of stared at her and was totally overcome with emotion. It was just looking at her and hardly believing that she's really ours" (A4). Katherine could not see Brett just after birth because she was just too tired and sleepy from the drugs, but the next morning she could not wait for the nurse to leave so that she could have a good look at her daughter. Brett was different than Katherine expected. Her dark hair, her face, her chubby cheeks were a big surprise. At this point Katherine was just curious, looking at her baby like an object to be examined. Susan, on the other hand, was not surprised by her baby's looks, "He came out looking how I had expected. I wasn't surprised" (S4). Earlier in pregnancy Susan had maintained that she had always thought her baby to be a separate person, so she was not surprised but just felt good about feeling him and seeing him. Jane's remarks, too, show her beginning relationship with Lisa as a separate being. "She opened her eyes and wasn't crying, and had a very good long look at both Jim and I, very intelligently, almost as if she recognized us by our voices or something. It's just so overwhelming . . . that you can't turn her down" (J3). Often women want to see the baby's face, to have face to face contact, to really see the child as a separate being, to look into the child's eyes. Eye contact with the infant may be a critical release during the first few hours (Seiden 1978: 85). The mother's response to the child is very much dependent on the infant's response to the mother.

Attachment

It is through the Otherness of the baby, and seeing that Otherness, that the woman begins to understand herself in relation to that person. "Little ancestor, sweet baby, how you temper me, deepen. Like an ancient smithy working slowly" (Chesler 1979: 281). One-for-the-Other starts with the cutting of the cord.

> So after he showed her to us he handed me the scissors and wanted me to cut the cord. I didn't want to. I wanted Jim to do it, but the doctor insisted I should cut it. Finally I did it but, boy, it was tough to cut, like a thick rope. (J3)

It is difficult cutting the cord—that irreparable cut—that accepts the infant as Other. For mothers it means changing with the needs of the child. The physical body processes of pregnancy and birth, as well as nursing, require the mother to accept constantly shifting definitions of herself. From being one, to being two. When one looks at and sees the child, there is no choice. As Jane said, "You can't turn her down."

When we think of Brenda's experience, when she turned away from her baby at birth—refusing to hold her and refusing to look at her—one wonders how her move to motherhood was made more difficult. Brenda recognized that she was holding back from looking at her child. She said, "I figured that she would be messy—red guck all over her, or some kind of discharge that would come down the birth canal with her. I didn't want to see a kid that was all yucky" (B3). Did her reluctance to look at her child retard her transformation to mother? Did her reluctance to accept the "guck" as well as her daughter's beauty make her progress to mothering more difficult? Brenda's response to her body in pregnancy as ugly and her distaste for the idea of the vernix and blood on her baby, may have distanced her from the bodily bond. Breastfeeding was also abhorrent to Brenda. "Thank goodness for formula," she said (B2). Did this bodily estrangement deny her a natural bridge to attentive love?

Separation

My son was perhaps four weeks old—how hard it is to remember dates and times you once thought you would never forget. I was nursing him every three or four hours. I was tired and had lain down for a nap. After a long sleep, I woke refreshed. Suddenly thoughts of my child rushed through my body—my breasts were painful and were starting to leak. But why had I not heard his cry? I was confused by this long sleep. I did not expect that I could have slept through his need for me. I found him in the garden contentedly sleeping in his carriage beside his father. His father had changed him and fed him with the breast milk that I had saved. Someone else could feed my baby! I was not always needed! My husband remembers that day, too. He found out that he could care for his child in a new way. Before that experience his care had been for us as mother/child, as one. Now he had a glimpse of his unique and personal relationship with his child. He had fed him. It was a turning point for both of us. A weaning from the mother and a bonding to the father. "Naturally" women nurture babies, "culturally" others can also be a part of this important task. This example shows a kind of dialectic of attachment and separation (Robert Burch, Personal Communication, May 17, 1986). First, there is the intrauterine bond and the separation of birth, for the sake of the I-Thou bond of mother and child; and, secondly, there is the separation of growing-maturing mother and child for the sake of a deeper I-Thou bond. Yet, both forms of separation are not simply something the mother/parents grant, the baby is born in its own time. The child gradually realizes adult freedom because the child wins it. Mothers and fathers begin to recognize more clearly the selfhood of the baby.

Christine, who from early pregnancy talked about her need to continue in her career, felt that she could be a good mother and still pursue her career. She said:

> There is quite a bit of challenge in combining the two. It is sobering thinking about the future, in maintaining my career and my relationship to my husband and child. And yet what I couldn't anticipate before was how important my child is to me and how strong that part of me is. (C6)

In fact, her mothering influences her work, and she thinks that is good. "I can't switch off who I am with my child. He is too much a part of me. How I relate to my husband and my child is where I get my ideas" (C6). Of course, it is not always easy for Christine, since both she and her husband want to be parents and have careers. Sometimes she thinks, "Better if I were a happy housewife," at the same time as knowing "that would be a disaster" (C7).

Katherine, in moving back to full-time work, said to her boss, "I have too much to do" (K5). She would never have said that before. Before Brett she would have come early or stayed late to get the work done. Now she is not prepared to do that. Her thoughts are directed to her child. She cannot ignore her relationship, her responsibility, to her child. The reality of a mother's attachment to her child and her work reinforces the chauvinistic prejudice about the reliability of women workers who are mothers. Instead of accepting that reality as negative, the work world may benefit by attention to "having children on one's mind." As more fathers take on the daily responsibilities of children, these negative attitudes may change.

For Anna, the first few weeks at work were the most difficult. She took a photograph to work with her which showed Jena pouting. It was just how Anna, herself, was feeling. The decision to go back to part-time work was not easy, but she knew that she too needed the stimulation of being "in the world." She did not want, as she said earlier, "for Bill to be her window to the world" (A2). She needed to have her own place. Brenda worried about being bored at home and went back to work about two months after Suzie was born. Susan talked about her need for adult companionship. Jane and Susan had difficulty thinking of someone looking after their children, as all the women did to some extent. But for Jane, her decision to be the primary parent in the ongoing care of Lisa was based on two factors. First, that her husband is "really very happy in the role of provider," and secondly, she felt that she could go back to her career when Lisa is older, "but I can never go back to the time when she's young and dependent" (J5).

It is necessary to reassess the notion that the woman as mother must be the prime caretaker of children and all that is involved in that role (Dinnerstein 1976; Chodorow 1978). Anna, Christine, and Susan talked, rather casually, about their husbands staying home to look after the child. Christine said that it was a possibility, but she wondered what she would miss if he should do that (C1). Although Bill liked the idea of staying home, Anna thought he was "romanticizing" it, especially in light of how demanding Jena really was to look after (A6). Susan thought that she would do better at home than Paul would. "I think that he would go nuts, he has to be doing things all the time—I don't think he would be happy at home. I do a lot more homey things. I sew and do crafts. I can teach the piano. But I wonder if I will be able to stay home without much adult contact" (S1). So, while there is ambivalence, it is usually women who stay with the child or make the arrangements about who will look after the child. Christine, Brenda, Katherine, and Anna searched out the neighbor, sister-in-law, mother, or the stranger who would care for their children while they returned to work.

Finding the right person was a problem for all of them except Brenda. Brenda had decided before the birth of Suzie that she would go back to work and had found a neighbor to care for her child. Because of her shift and weekend work, it was often Tom, her husband, who would baby-sit. Tom's use of the word "baby-sit" indicates his relationship to the job of caring for his child—a word often used by fathers, rarely by mothers.

Although the children had taken some time to adjust to the arrangement of child care, each mother thought that her child had benefitted in some way from it—being with other children or learning different ways of doing things. Each woman felt that the time spent away from the child made her more able to give to the child when she was home.

Christine spoke at length about her child care arrangements because although her time was flexible at graduate school she had considerable pressures that had to be met. One of her advisors had accused her of "putting her child at risk" which, she said, if she had not been so sure of herself, would have brought her to tears. She felt that he, as a male, did not understand her need to do what she was doing, and, of course, would not question a new father in the same position (C7).

Yet, the problem of child care is a real one in today's society. Some feel that there should be more and better day care, even universal day care. Others feel that no day care can solve the problem of the child's need for a home and the freedom from institutional restraints that the home provides. Again we need to ask, what is so important about a home? A home is a place where one can be oneself, where one is accepted for oneself. It is also the place where there is a mother, a father, grandparents, or other people who are devoted to the child in an "irrational" way, made possible by unconditional love. While there are no perfect parents, no perfect home, the place where a child can gain the basic foundation of human life may best be found in the home within the fold of loving parents.

MINDING THE TIME

"Days are full of doing things," said Jane, "but nothing gets done" (J5). The world of a woman as mother gets turned upside down in unpredictable ways. Chicago's image of the faceless lady expressed the price women pay as nurturers—"as trapped by the needs of those one gives life to" (1985: 92, 96). Chronic fatigue, disorganization, multitudinous commitments, guilt, a fragmented existence all come with the nourishing requirements of the Other, the child. It was what Christine was worried about, "You see, work is manageable, you know what you can do, you organize" (C1). She saw women at her work who appeared fatigued and harassed who claimed they had trouble trying to accomplish all they needed to do. How does one organize the time with a new baby as responsibility?

They say to be there at eight, so you try to be there by that time, which may not necessarily fit in with the way she would normally be doing things. (K4)

I think I am still organized to a degree, and I think about things ahead of time. When I start making dinner, it's two in the afternoon, when he's settled down because I know that at supper time he is up. I just take advantage of the time I have. (S5)

If you want to have sex, we have to do it now because it is twenty to ten and the baby is asleep. "Whatever happened to spontaneous lovemaking?" (C4)

Living with a child changes one's relationship to time. Instead of hours and minutes, work time, coffee time, or dinner time, etc., the days are broken into sleep time, feeding time, bathing time, and laundry time. It may seem endless, and one wonders if one can live through it. There is never enough time for sleep. There is not much time for oneself, as mother.

How can we give enough time to children? We hear about full-time mothers, part-time mothers, latch-key children, and even the notion of quality versus quantity time. Valerie Polakow Suransky (1982) in her book *The Erosion of Childhood* looked at the institutions that are set up to care for children. Here we see slotted time for children: going to the bathroom time, eating lunch time, cleaning up time, and so on. Where is the freedom of play time, doing nothing time, and private time, that we all, especially children, need?

SPACE FOR THE CHILD AND THE MOTHER

Giving birth changes how you see the world. You know, when I walk down the street I see each person being born. I exist in relation to human vulnerability and nakedness as never before. (Chesler 1979: 191)

"I Know How Babies Are Now"

Both Susan and Anna remarked on how they see the world, especially other children, differently now. "It is hard to see parents who are mean to children, or even think of the fact that some mothers put their child on a four-hour schedule" (S6). "When I see a child on television, it is like seeing my child. I see all children as my child," said Anna (A6). She talked of the earthquake in Mexico where babies were found in the rubble days later. It is the knowing—"what babies are like now," and imagining them crying and crying, all alone—that moved her. She does not think she would have responded with such emotion before Jena's birth—and she thinks it has added a dimension to her life that she sees as good.

Yet Anna wants a happy balance between emotion and reason. Although she is happy for her new "softness," as she calls it, being touched by small animals, being more cuddly, with more need for closeness, she wants to be part of the larger reasoning world as well. Katherine, too, said, "I had to make myself watch the news so that I would know what is going on in the world" (K5). In the recognition that

> Passions of maternity are so sudden, intense, and confusing . . . we often remain ignorant of the perspective, the thought, that is developed from mothering. . . . Intellectual activities are distinguishable but not separable from disciplines of feeling. There is a unity of reflection, judgment, and emotion. This unity I call "maternal thinking" (Ruddick 1983: 213–14).

The "child on my mind," then is a way of being, and not merely an emotional reaction to children. It is a way of being and thinking about and experiencing the world—the world as a good place for children. Anna, earlier in pregnancy, wondered if this is true—if the world *is* a good place for children. She said:

> I get so frustrated with people who tell us all the horror stories about children. We were out for dinner and all they could talk about was how bratty kids were. I thought, "Why bother, why have kids?" "Don't tell me this stuff, I don't care to hear it." I think a lot of times that this world doesn't cater to children. There is a certain amount of prejudice against children. I know you have to change your life, but [one must] change it to the benefit of both. (A3)

Germaine Greer (1984) points out that within our society the world of the "adult" and the world of the "child" are becoming more distant and unequal. In a society that does not tend to value children, as children, it may be easy to put one's child out of one's mind. In a society that esteems public work, that continually strives for better material goods, that discounts child care with its low wages and low prestige, it may be easy for the woman once "fragmented by the child on her mind" to accept society's dominant goals in her search for self worth. But the child needs a mother, and a father too. Who will mother the child?

"I Know How Mothers Are Now"

The mother needs the child. In her recent book *The Anatomy of Freedom* (1984: 192, 196), Morgan writes about an international conference held in 1980. Here, she says "ordinary folks" from local women's organizations, feminist alternative media, and women's religious, health, and community groups gather together to talk. Here an Iraqi refugee told an American Jewish feminist that her eleven-year-old son has just been sentenced to five years at hard labor by the Saddam Hussein regime. "My God, my son is just that age," replied the American woman. They weep in each others arms. Mothers know how mothers are—how mothers need their children. They weep in recognition of the pain of seeing a world that has lost sight of the child as child. Living side-by-side children, having our mind attuned to children, prompts increasingly reflective questions—we begin to doubt ourselves and feel guilty. Did I do right? Am I doing right? As we are transformed to mother we are forced to question ourselves.

To have one's mind full of thoughts of the child—while it may at times fragment thinking—pays respect to the child and its needs, and enriches the parents' life. It causes one to think of the nature of the world, a world as a community for children.

Chapter 8

The Relationship of Knowledge to Self-Understanding

In Chapters 3 through 7, I explored the transformative moments (themes) that women experience as they become mothers. These moments—the decision to have a child, the experienced presence of the child (I-Thou relationship), the separation of that experienced presence through pain that can lead to integration and wholeness, the appropriation of responsibility for oneself and the world as one accepts the presence of the child, and the "mindfulness" to the child that occurs with a child in one's life—are not stages or steps in a process. The notion of "moments" encompasses an enlarged view of experience, unifying the two words "momentous" and "momentary" (O'Brien 1981: 47). This is a view that goes beyond the linear approach to encompass a notion of the hermeneutic circle, a concept that shows increasing depth of understanding as one again and again faces a previous theme of one's lived experience. The moments of transformation, as hermeneutically revealed, may even be seen as a hologram in which the "part is as great as the sum—or the part *is*, in fact, the sum." To illustrate:

the moment of the decision to bring a child into one's life, in itself, shows the transformative experience. Yet the presence of the child in the mother's body interacts with that decision to deepen and intensify it. Or, within the moment of decision, a decision beyond the rational, comes responsibility. Or as the presence of the child is experienced in different ways, the separation becomes possible, and, indeed necessary, and through separation comes the overwhelming experience of having a child on one's mind, in day-to-day, worldly ways. Thus, transformative moments through hermeneutic encounter do not fragment in linear or categorical ways the wholeness of the childbirth experience, but reveal the depth, the profoundness, the complexity, and, indeed, the perplexity, that "becoming a mother" offers women.

APPROACHES TO CHILDBIRTH KNOWLEDGE

Recall Gail and Christine from Chapter 1. They gave birth under the influence of differing approaches to childbirth knowledge. There is need to analyze the underlying forms of knowledge that lead to particular individual application. Such an analysis places the forms of knowledge in the foreground so that one is able to see what is at stake, that is, what interests privilege particular approaches to knowledge. Such an analysis needs to explore both the *strengths* and *problems* associated with the various approaches to childbirth knowledge.

Any analysis comes from within a frame of reference, a way of thinking, which one cannot step outside. We belong to a tradition and are shaped by that tradition. It is important, then, to acknowledge that this analysis finds its root in a critical thinking arising from personal knowledge of women's situation in this culture, a world which upholds patriarchal attitudes—placing great value on objectivity, rationality, development, progress, efficiency, expediency, and technology. Therefore, the effort will attempt to go beyond documentation or reiteration of chronological facts of history. It will also go beyond attacking and rejecting these knowledge traditions, or even taking sides, for that blinds one to what is at stake. Rather the approach aims to "be responsible for the world of tradition" in which we are situated (Arendt 1961). The challenge, for me, and for the reader, is to appropriate tradition while being critically aware of the modes of thought that constitute the tradition, and then to articulate a just and viable tradition more appropriate to our present situation (Ruether 1983; Elshtain 1982).

Present approaches to childbirth knowledge can be categorized in the following way: obstetrical, midwifery, methodological and critical. At present, obstetrical knowledge is the foundation of maternity care to which the other forms of knowledge have responded. Midwifery knowledge, while once the backbone of care, is now making a resurgence as it is being shown to be a knowledge form that is valuable to women. The "how-to" approach within obstetrical and midwifery traditions gives practical skills and tools to the childbearing woman to help her handle her individual labor. The category designated critical approach questions obstetrical, methodological, and midwifery knowledge from a number of viewpoints, including social, technological, and feminist perspectives.

The Obstetrical View

Strengths. The science of obstetrics has brought safety to the childbirth experience. Mortality rates show a dramatic decrease in recent years. The perinatal mortality rate in Canada of 20–30 per 1000 in 1970 is now close to 10 per 1000; the rate of infant death in one major Canadian city decreased from a rate of 48.9 per 1000 in 1930 (ELBH 1984) to 9.0 per 1000 in 1985 (EBH 1985). Health and safety of the mother and baby are the foundational factors underlying the management of childbirth practice in Canada.

Development of technology and the emphasis placed on scientific research in medicine have played an important role in this move to safe childbirth. Ultrasound is used as a diagnostic tool in pregnancy to assess the growth of the fetus, to search for abnormalities (such as a pelvic mass), or to identify problems with the placenta, etc. It is also used in fetal monitors which have made it possible for experts in major centers to give advice to practitioners in rural hospitals (Tucker 1979). Episiotomies are performed to prevent unnecessary tearing of perineal tissues during delivery, to prevent loss of tone in the pelvic muscle, and to prevent damage to the newborn by shortening the second stage of labor (Thacker and Banta 1983). Artificial rupture of the membranes, drugs, and forceps are used to assist and/or initiate the process of labor. The incidence of cesarean sections, now considered a safe surgical procedure, has greatly increased in the last ten years, from 4–6 percent in 1974 to 15–17 percent in 1982 (even to 30 percent in some tertiary care hospitals) (Elkins 1983: 2). In some situations, it is said, that in the search for the "perfect" baby, women are beginning to choose cesarean births to avoid the risk to the baby of vaginal births (K2).

Scientific obstetrics takes place in hospitals where medical experts with access to sophisticated equipment stand near at hand to respond immediately to any problem that may arise. At present over 97 percent of women in Canada and the United States have hospital births. Women are encouraged to be active in the early stages of labor and are often placed in the lithotomy position with the use of stirrups for delivery. This allows the doctor access to the perineal area in order to perform the episiotomy, to use forceps, and to employ other maneuvers if the necessity arises. Flexibility of birthing position has developed in some hospitals to include the semi-sitting position, and the birthing chair. Sterile technique used to prevent infection carries with it the admonition, as to Jane, "to look but not touch" as the baby is born. Procedures such as intravenous infusion, enema, perineal shave, and attachment of the fetal monitor, vary from being initiated routinely to being used only in selected cases, depending on the skills and preferences of the doctor. The science of obstetrics approaches childbirth as a process to be initiated and monitored so that the course and outcome can be carefully controlled (Böhme 1984).

As with any knowledge form that becomes very specific and technical, knowledge used in the management of childbirth has become confined to experts, the doctors and hospital staff (Berger and Luckmann 1967: 79–92). Such knowledge is controlled and legitimized from within, in that professional groups develop their own methodology and logic to insure safe practice. For example, in 1981 the Alberta College of Physicians and Surgeons banned physicians from attending births at home in the interests of safety, thus limiting the possibilities for having professional medical support at births outside of the hospital.

Scientific, technological knowledge of childbirth has gained rapid support since the turn of the century which led to a move from home to hospital care and from care given by a midwife to care by a family doctor and obstetrician (Wertz and Wertz 1979; Ehrenreich and English 1979; Barrington 1985, chap. 2; Shorter 1982). So universal is the acceptance of medical opinion that many women have come to understand it as the absolute truth. Fundamental trust is placed in the doctor. Some women say gratefully, "We owe the lives of our children to them." Others say, "The experience for me doesn't matter as long as my baby is healthy." or "One forgets the pain." Obstetrical knowledge is now the common, taken-for-granted approach expected by most women. Reliance on the doctor as the carrier of that knowledge is sensed in Christine's comment just after being admitted to hospital. "They got me comfortable," she said, "Dr. Henry was on the floor. I heard his voice right away, and I guess he had had another baby, and that was very comforting" (C3).

Problems. Comforting, yes, . . . and yet? On August 26, 1985, Canada's national radio open-line show asked its listeners to respond to the question, "Should doctors be the only ones to deliver babies?" The question, itself, is a curious one. O-lan had no one with her—she gave birth to her child alone. Nowadays, women want and expect someone to help them. The problem comes with the helper. Does the helper take over the process so extensively that she or he "has" the baby? Is this loss of status of women as reproducers due to the fact that women have lost the knowledge once available to them to trust their own bodies? Or is it because women have accepted the underlying opinion that a medicalized birth is safe, and therefore give themselves over to that expertise and authority? Or, conversely, could it be that the separation of birth from the social context has led to a situation where childbirth is, in one sense, outside women's domain?

Other voices also suggest that there are problems related to obstetrical knowledge. Women are saying that certain procedures such as the perineal shave is degrading, some say that the hospital is cold and mechanized, and some say that the dependency on medical specialists is disabling. As early as 1974, Doris Haire challenged current medical practices, such as the routine use of drugs, the hospital as a suitable environment, ambivalent breastfeeding counseling, separating mothers and babies at birth, and many other routine practices. Her challenge has been heard and yet there are still routine practices that have not been carefully researched. While women agreed that safety is important, they began to question how safety can be considered outside of the whole context and meaning of giving birth (Arms 1975; Kitzinger and Davis 1978; Rothman 1982). Some began to question the notion that hospitals (the best location for implementation of obstetrical knowledge) provide the safest environment for childbirth (Mehl, Peterson, Whitt and Hawes 1977; Stewart and Stewart 1976). Countries, such as the Netherlands or Sweden, which employ midwives and which have a high percentage of home births, show lower infant mortality rates than countries like Canada where midwives are not recognized legally and home births are rare (Barrington 1985: 124). In fact, the problem of safety has not been carefully researched; and until that research is carried out, there is no conclusive evidence from which to evaluate safety of hospital births in contrast to home births (Hoff and Schneiderman 1985).

Iatrogenic disease, not included in indices of mortality, is, according to Dr. Caldero Barcia, former head of the International Confederation of Gynaecology & Obstetrics, "the main cause of fetal distress" (quoted in Barrington 1985: 122). Hospital births, with access to technological tools, are subject to hazards which are not always nor easily identified. In the hospital there is a greater chance for a woman to encounter an episiotomy, the use of forceps, cesarean section, and other interventions raising the possibility of complications (Young 1987). The fetal monitor is a case in point. Baumgarten (1981) defended his position of recommending fetal monitoring for all women in labor by showing a relationship between increased use of fetal monitoring and lower mortality rates. The research by Haverkamp, Thompson, McFee, and Cetrulo, however, did not support this recommendation. In fact, Haverkamp et al. stated that routine monitoring is unnecessary or potentially harmful, citing the striking increase in cesarean sections performed for fetal distress in the group of women attached to the fetal monitor (1976: 316). While scientific research has not demonstrated any harmful effects from the use of ultrasound in childbirth, neither has there been conclusive support to show the certainty of its safety (ICEA 1983). Like many other exciting and innovative technological possibilities, the fetal monitor was used without the benefit of careful research (Young 1983). Barrington (1985: 128–29) outlined the chain of interventive events that begin with the innocuous routine administration of intravenous fluids which lead to confinement to bed, drug administration to stimulate the uterus, forceps, lithotomy position, and episiotomy. Brackbill, Rice, and Young, in *Birth Trap* (1984), argued convincingly that there are risks with any technological intervention, however innocuous. It is also true that interventions in labor and delivery reflect cyclical changes in medical and social opinion rather than medical research (Wolkind and Zajicek 1981: 126).

Childbirth management, on the part of both doctors and nurses, shows vividly the interests at stake (Rothman 1982). "Management" means to direct or control, to make submissive to one's authority or discipline. Of course "management" is not necessarily a negative term. We use expressions such as "one manages one's own life." But in the scientific context of the management of childbirth the word "management" implies a situation directed by doctors, nurses, or even machines (such as the fetal monitor described in Christine's situation). Management, as control, is expressed in terms of mortality rates (control over death) and in terms of the initiation and control of stages of labor within predetermined time frames (control over women's bodies). Indeed, control can be a desirable quality, but there is a need to question who controls whom, how, and why.

Let us explore the medical and technical power over death we have come to accept. According to Oakley (1979, 1980b), the prevention of death seen in perinatal and maternal mortality rates remains the chief yardstick by which obstetricians judge the value of their work. We have a situation, then, where "keeping people alive has become the primary medical goal and the quality of the lives thus extended has seemed a secondary consideration" (Oakley 1980b: 27). Illich (1976), Oakley (1980b), and others have carefully analyzed the notion that decreasing mortality rates are directly attributable to the impact of medicine, or in this case, to obstetrical care. While there is a rise of modern professional and technological expertise at the same time as lowered mortality and morbidity rates, it is false to assume a cause/effect relationship. Possible contributing factors to the lowered mortality rates are higher maternal age and lower parity, improved nutrition, availability of effective contraceptives, changing abortion laws, decreased use of tobacco and alcohol by pregnant women, environmental improvement in water supplies, sewage disposal, and housing, increased knowledge of the childbirth process by parents, as well as the choice women now have as to whether or not to have children at all. There is also the clash between the index of statistical survival and many mothers' own assessment of reproductive success. "Women evaluate the success of their childbirths in a more holistic way than the medical frame of reference allows," said Oakley (1980b: 27).

The very fact that pregnancies are termed high- or low-risk already places women in a battle against death—a central issue. The continuum of risk, knowing there is always risk, is problematic. "Discovering that one is in a high-risk group increases the risk" (Benner 1985: 13). Then, too, women who are initially defined as low risk may be moved along the continuum to high-risk when treated with the measures that are appropriate for use with the high-risk patient. Knowledge used to care for women who are ill or diseased during pregnancy and labor may be inappropriate to the well childbearing woman, and introducing obstetrical knowledge into her care may move her along the path to becoming "at risk," for "each technical, chemical or surgical intervention carries its own risk" (Barrington 1985: 122). A simple example may clarify this notion. If a laboring woman is put to bed, and placed on her back because of the fetal monitor, she may need medication to control her pain which would otherwise be dealt with by her own move-ment—standing, rocking, or walking. The medication may lead to further interventions, stimulation of labor through rupture of the membranes or drugs—the chain effect.

Most obstetrical "patients" are not ill and do not require medical treatment at all. The problem then becomes one of balancing the benefits and hazards to two different populations of mothers and babies, those who need medical care and those who do not (Oakley 1980b: 26). Because risk is a fact of life and one can never be sure, it is almost necessary, under the umbrella of obstetrical knowledge, for an obstetrician to say that it is necessary to start an intravenous infusion on all patients "just in case" (Brackbill et al. 1984). This attitude is, of course, partly due to the increasing number of litigations. To "take a chance," when it means to take a chance with life, especially the life of a child, is not acceptable. The problem with litigation is that the capacity for judgment, that intellectual rationality, has dominated the power of judgment, which is a moral activity (Bollnow 1987). The more we are bound by the rationality of litigations the more we lose the moral judgment powerful enough to make human choices.

The problems of obstetrical knowledge become clearer when one begins to question its premise as "truth." Scientific research, the foundation of obstetrical knowledge, which restricts the number of intervening variables so as to discover basic and functional relationships, is unimpeded by situa-tional details (Franklin 1984). Knowledge that separates itself from the every-day life of peoples' experience (in the effort to maintain ultimate objectivity), needs care in its practical application. It becomes easy to gear technology for use "as intended" (it is available, therefore it should be used), rather than be concerned about its use in the "right" situation. It is easy to see how women may begin to feel like machines when, in a technological environ-ment, they are attached to various pieces of equipment. For the woman, such an environment can be an alienating experience, which has the danger of stripping the childbirth of meaning for women (Green 1985).

There has been a response on the part of the obstetrical team to the grumbling voices of expectant mothers and fathers, and the childbirth ad-vocates (some being the experts themselves). Efforts are being made to hu-manize obstetrical care through family-centered initiatives which include informing women of their choices, designing home-like birthing rooms, building free-standing birth centers, or implementing other programs, such as the Single Unit Delivery System, which provide opportunities for the women to labor, deliver, and to spend the postpartum period in the same room (McKay 1982). Another recent idea is for expectant parents to prepare a Birth Plan which lists their preferences of childbirth management which they discuss with their care givers and which they take with them to hospital at the time of labor (Simkin et al. 1984: 12–13).

The remarkable strides made in saving lives, especially of very ill babies and mothers, makes it difficult to question the appropriateness of a medical science approach. Even the humanizing procedures can be seen as appeasing the concerns of childbearing women by "giving them what they want" while maintaining control of the birthing process. Then again, one wonders if the knowledge and practice of childbirth should not be "human" in the first place. Thus we see that while obstetrical knowledge has been useful in improving the physical safety of mothers and babies, there are problems with basing the childbirth experience exclusively on its scientific foundation. Concern has been expressed that obstetrical and technical knowledge, by seeing birth in such a narrow focus, puts into jeopardy the quality of human experience.

The Midwifery View

Strengths. One day, a few years ago, I stayed with a friend during her planned home birth attended by professional midwives who worked closely with a doctor in the city where I live. This is what I remember: Richard called me at six on that bright, clear May morning to say that Paula had been in labor since about three. Alice, the midwife, had been called, and Bill was coming to look after the children, Candace, age seven, and Paul, age five. Richard's mother was making breakfast when I arrived. I spent the day with Paula as she dealt with her frequent, painful contractions. Sometimes she sat on the living room floor supported by Richard; sometimes she walked to the bathroom, stopping frequently and leaning on us for support while the contraction passed; and sometimes she lay in the soothing water of a warm bath. Sometimes the house rang with laughter, and sometimes the quiet permeated the rooms to support her rest. As the "pains" became more intense, the tension of the family was evident. The children asked Bill to take them to the store. The grandmother quietly stood in the bedroom doorway, the tension written on her face. The midwives made periodic checks and waited. Richard and I stayed close to Paula. As we acknowledged her pain and her strength, she took hold. She needed to be reminded that she could do it. Baby Joanna was born in the late afternoon, within the presence of her family and friends, and was immediately taken into the arms of her tired mother where she nursed at her breast. In a short time, the baby was immersed in a warm bath surrounded and admired by her father, sister, and brother. Later, we all gathered around the table for a feast to celebrate the birth, to celebrate the child, and to celebrate the mother.

Paula just could not think of having her third child in the hospital under the influence of obstetrical knowledge. What she feared was the sterile atmosphere, the attitude of doctors and nurses which she found debilitating, the separation from her other children and friends, the drugs and procedures, and her overwhelming fear of the pain. So while obstetrical knowledge strives to reduce or eliminate pain, Paula's fear of pain was increased within an environment supported by the application of obstetrical knowledge. She and Richard wanted this birth to be in their own hands as they had begun to question the shortcomings of the medical birth and its notion of safety. They had read the abundant material coming out of the childbirth movement, the women's movement, and the political movement which put into question the very roots of medicalized childbirth.

Paula did not have an episiotomy this time. From my nursing experience I was astounded to watch the delivery of the baby's head as it was guided so slowly (I thought) over the intact perineum by the hands of the midwife. All the births that I had seen were rapid by comparison as the baby's head was easily delivered through the incised perineal tissues. The benefits of episiotomies have not been well researched, but the effects experienced by women are well documented. Pain (for five months, C5), edema, and infection are the primary risks (Thacker and Banta 1983; Barrington 1985). There was hard labor pain for Paula, pain as strong as with her other two births, but she lived through it with less distress as she moved around her own house with the support of those who loved her.

Midwifery knowledge has been practiced since the beginning of time and is recognized as a legitimate and necessary profession in most countries. At the present time 75 percent of the world's population is born with the assistance of midwives within the home, the hospital, or the birth center. "Of the two hundred and ten countries in the World Health Organization, only eight, including Canada, are without systematic provision for support by a midwife during a normal birth" (NDP 1983: 16). Midwifery knowledge takes two distinct forms, traditional or lay midwifery and the "new," professional midwifery. In Canada, the move from the traditional midwife (also called lay healer, or wise woman) to the professional midwife occurred over the last hundred years (Barrington 1985: 35). The decline of traditional midwifery knowledge and practice was due to the rise of a male-dominated medical profession (and its need for economic security), the push toward hospital birth where midwives were not welcome, and the emerging nursing profession which supported hospital maternity care (Barrington 1985: 25–32; Wertz and Wertz 1979). Benoit (1984) contends that it was modern professional midwives who were the main medical actresses in the historical struggle to "scientize" and regulate midwifery practice in Canada, particularly in places like Newfoundland which has a long tradition of lay midwifery. The well-meaning actions of these male medical professionals and the professional midwives cannot, of course, be discounted.

The traditional midwife, still practicing in many parts of the world (Jordan

1980), gains her knowledge through observation, personal experience, and through oral and craft traditions handed on from woman to woman, often from mother to daughter. The language of midwifery knowledge is the everyday vernacular and, therefore, available to everyone. Prerequisites of her role are experience, maturity, good character, and an intense knowledge of the local culture and people (Benoit 1984; Böhme 1984). The midwife's task was to help the birth event take its own course, watching, waiting, and assisting the woman to bear the child—to bear what nature would bring. "Birth was nature in the sense of the Greek concept of *physis*: nature is what takes its own course, that which unfolds, reveals itself" (Böhme, p. 380). This knowledge respects the rhythm of women's bodies to bring the child to birth. As traditional midwives are women, their knowledge was self-knowledge, which is a subjective knowing of the experience of childbirth. Benoit (1984) suggested that the traditional midwife, the holder of lived-world knowledge (Chamberlain 1981, calls it old wife's knowledge), and today's professional midwives, whose knowledge can be said to be the art and science of childbirth, are very distinct in actual practice. According to Böhme (1984), in industrial countries traditional midwifery knowledge, knowledge of childbirth as a biographical and social event, has been lost; and with the loss of knowledge, the event itself has disappeared.

The present practice of midwifery, seen in the professional midwife and developed out of traditional midwifery, provides continuing care for the woman over the pregnancy, birth, and early postpartum period. Professional midwifery focusses on the normal, that is, the well woman's experience of birth. In fact, these new midwives are specialists in uncomplicated childbirth. Their training, as distinct from medical and nursing training, provides comprehensive knowledge on all aspects of normal birth (physiological, social, and emotional). Midwifery knowledge provides education about nutrition, labor and delivery, preparation for the actual birth, pregnancy surveillance (routine checks of weight, urinary glucose and protein, blood pressure, and other routine laboratory work), and postpartum care. Regular contact between the midwife and mother throughout pregnancy is focussed around diet, exercise, health habits, home life, and emotional concerns. The midwife meets the woman early in, or even prior to, pregnancy and continues the contact through to the postpartum period. This continuous support, essential during labor and delivery, develops over time by knowing the woman, her situation, and her wishes and, optimally, results in a relationship of mutual respect and trust. The trust established through this continuity of care is felt necessary for a healthy birth. The underlying focus of midwifery knowledge is, then, to support the birthing mother and newborn child and to create a situation where the mother, father, and baby can share the first moments together. The midwives are in a sense "women helpers" rather than "doctor's assistants" as nurses have been seen (Jordan 1980).

Only recently in Canada have midwives begun to work as midwives in some hospitals and in free-standing birth centers, as well as in the home. Most often the midwives work as nurses on obstetrical units. However, not all of the new midwives are nurses, and some feel that nursing education with its emphasis on disease is neither appropriate nor necessary for midwives. Like nurses, most professional midwives are female, and that fact is felt by some to be an important element in creating the understanding needed between the childbearing woman and her care givers. "The wisdom and compassion a woman can intuitively experience in childbirth can make her a source of healing and understanding for other women," said Gaskin (1977: 11), the self-trained midwife from The Farm. One thinks of the Greek goddess of childbearing, Artemis, who, although childless herself, decreed that only those who had given birth and were past the childbearing age could be midwives. The self-understanding that midwives have about their own birth-giving bodies may provide a thoughtfulness that an objective male view cannot bridge.

Problems. Yet, there are questions about midwifery knowledge. The acknowledged distinction between traditional or lay midwifery and professional midwifery makes one question if there is any substantial difference between professional midwifery knowledge and obstetrical knowledge. Is not professional midwifery knowledge just less expert and therefore second best? While it appears that midwifery knowledge is distinct, it may be that both it and obstetrical knowledge operate within the same framework, in a hierarchical relationship. Medicine's influence has become so complex and all encompassing that many life events are now part of medical practices and treatments as evidenced by pre-pregnancy counseling for girls or the treatment of menopause as disease (Donoff and Paton 1984; MacPherson 1981).

But, what if Joanna had died in childbirth? What if the midwives' knowledge could not handle the emergency that no one could predict? There is no emergency back-up for midwife-attended home births other than sudden transfer to the hospital. At the present time, with all the scientific and technological advances, matters of safety, relief of debilitating pain, expediency, and efficiency cannot be ignored. Although statistics show that home births may be safe for those women who are not ill and whose unborn babies are growing well, there is the problem of never knowing for sure whether complications at birth will develop. What about the unexpected maternal hemorrhage, for example? Although the midwife carries with her oxygen and drugs to treat hemorrhage, this may not be enough.

The medical profession stands strongly against midwife-attended home births. It appears reluctant to give up their position and income (which has been called "economic territorialism," Barrington 1985; Brackbill et al. 1984) to share with midwives their present role in the hospital environment. According to the British Columbia Medical Association, the creation of the profession of nurse-midwifery would be a "regressive measure." The reluctance to consider midwifery knowledge as different and essential for the childbearing woman keeps it in the realm of second best: useful only if the woman and child are risk free (which, of course, is never a possibility— there is always risk).

Another consideration is the fact "that risks of hospital births are socially acceptable and the risks at home are not," said Murray Enkin, professor of obstetrics and gynecology, McMaster University (reported in Barrington 1985: 131). Rothman, too, acknowledged that "it is the profession of medicine which has been granted professional autonomy, the right to make decisions, and thus the right to make mistakes in childbirth management" (1985: 93). Anna and Bill acknowledged that they would be publicly censored if their baby should have problems in the home situation (A2). The parents and the professional midwives would be seen as—irresponsible, killers, murderers— while the staff in hospital would have been seen as "trying their best." Our society tries to push away death to the extent that some individuals (especially infants and elderly) are forced to live (sometimes even for research purposes) without any chance for a reasonably acceptable quality of life (Colen 1986; McDermott 1986; Chinn 1979). As a society we have accepted the medical view of childbirth management and can be critical of the practice of the alternative views.

Some have argued that it is selfish and morally wrong for women to be so preoccupied with their own needs that they take a chance with a midwife-attended birth. These people, including parents and specialists, say that in the interests of the baby it is not ethically right to take any chance if there is any risk to the baby (Hoff and Schneiderman 1985). Some have even charged that having a home birth is potentially a form of child abuse (Barrington 1985: 131). The massive increase in interventionist medical procedures in the last forty years have been in the interest of the baby (Shorter 1982). Fetal monitoring, episiotomy, cesarean section, and even forceps ultimately are meant to serve the health of the newborn baby. How could one not take all necessary precautions when a newborn is involved? Conversely, if midwifery knowledge is distinct and valuable for the childbearing woman, why should not the "high-risk" woman also be given the right to the midwife's knowledge and care. Relegating midwifery knowledge to "alternative" status limits the possibility of making it available to all women, those with no apparent problems as well as those designated high-risk. This concern forces examination of the very foundations of obstetrical and midwifery knowledge.

There are those who feel that midwifery knowledge is good because it is a way of reducing the spiralling cost of health care. It has been demonstrated that midwifery care, especially in the home setting or in a free-standing birth center is more economical than the technologically equipped hospital birth (Brackbill et al 1984; Barrington 1985; NDP 1983). Of course, it is necessary to contain and reduce the costs of health care, but the cost factor as a reason for the implementation of midwifery knowledge is problematic. There is the danger of people being treated differentially according to economic circumstances. The reason for using a particular form of knowledge needs to be assessed from the point of what is appropriate for good health and not from the ability to pay.

The Methodological View

Strengths. In the 1930s Grantly Dick-Read initiated the "how-to" movement in preparation for childbirth. Dick-Read and his followers, Lamaze in the 1950s, Bradley and Leboyer in the 1970s, and Odent in the 1980s, are medical doctors who developed techniques to reduce or remove pain for women (Lamaze and Bradley), reduce the trauma to the infant (Leboyer), and tap into the natural (primal) abilities of women (Odent). Dick-Read explored the relationship between tension and pain and applied it to childbirth. Women were encouraged to relax so that they could break the vicious circle of tension—pain—more tension—more pain. Lamaze based his work in psychoprophylaxis (or mind preparation) on Pavlov's theory of conditioned-response which called for women to learn to respond to the uterine contraction by active relaxation of muscular tension and to initiate a particular breathing pattern. Very specific in methodology, the Lamaze method teaches the woman to control her own childbirth experience not just by passive relaxation but by active decontraction in a very deliberate effort to have her mind control her body and to pattern her breathing to recognizable stages of labor. Bradley's fame centered around his concern for the active role of the father in controlled childbirth. The Bradley method, using a breathing pattern different from Lamaze, calls for the husband to act as coach throughout pregnancy and labor within the obstetrical milieu.

The increased interest in the well-being of the fetus and newborn is behind the work of Leboyer who described birth as a traumatic event for the baby. His efforts were directed to providing an environment conducive to welcoming the newborn into the world in a gentle, soothing way by dimming the delivery room lights, decreasing unnecessary noise, immersing the newborn in a warm bath, and giving gentle and stimulating massage to the baby. Leboyer claimed that by reducing the trauma to the newborn, the child would grow up happier, more intelligent, and physically stronger.

Odent, a strong critic of medicalized childbirth, has turned full circle and suggested that women themselves should be in charge of birthing. Odent, a male and a surgeon, attempted to demonstrate that women, primordially, know how to deliver their own babies and has been instrumental in creating a hospital environment which supports this innate ability. While revolutionary in nature, with no use of forceps, few episiotomies, a low cesarean section rate, and no pain relieving drugs, Odent's approach has caught the attention of childbearing women and childbirth activists but has done little to turn around every day practices in many Canadian hospitals.

If we are to meet the challenge from such ardent evangelists as Leboyer and Odent we must eliminate from our routines those things which are unnecessary and promote aspects which they emphasize, *within the bounds of sensible and safe obstetrics* (Romney and White 1984: 74).

Any substantial change in not contemplated.

There is, however, more to the methodological approach and the child-birth reform movement than indicated by the work of these famous medical men. Women have taken the lead in childbirth education for many years. Their energies have often been triggered by personal experience in childbirth, recognizing the need to share with other women their realization that child-birth is an experience to be enjoyed and treasured as active participants. Gaskin (1977), Kitzinger (1979b), Peterson (1981), Simkin et al. (1984), and Panuthos (1984) have developed, broadened, and surpassed the "guru" meth-odologies in an effort to educate women and men for childbirth.

Edwards and Waldorf revealed and clarified the male domination of child-birth. They said, "Even in the women's world of birthing babies we see innovation and reform dominated by the names of male obstetricians, while methods originated or developed by nurses, physical therapists, or midwives if they survive at all, are known by the name of whichever medical man made them famous" (1984: vii). In their book, *Reclaiming Birth*, the authors described childbirth heroines such as Margaret Gamper, Elisabeth Bing, Lester Hazell, Niles Newton, Doris Haire, Sheila Kitzinger, and Raven Lang who have struggled "to dignify the ordinary experience of women as they become mothers" (1984: xi), yet who are not as readily recognized as the famous males. Odent's (1984a: 118) statement that it is "time for male obstetricians would do well to progressively retire and restore childbirth to women," may not have much support from his obstetrical colleagues.

Recently developed breathing techniques and methods (within the last fifty years) have been based on the separation of mind and body. Such techniques of concentration to discipline the mind (hypnosis and muscle relaxation) are used to divert attention from the body as a way of controlling the pain and act like drugs which numb the mind to sensations of the body. Control of the mind over the body can separate the woman from the sensation of her labor, its pain or pleasure, its struggle and power. Mind control separates women from "being there." In contrast to this mind-body sepa-ration, imagery, symbolism, and breathing in response to the body's rhythm accept the integration of mind and body to assist the woman to give birth to the baby. Rather than using the breathing to control the pain, the breathing helps to relax the body to feel the pains (contractions), to go with them, to open oneself to the rhythm and wisdom of one's own body.

I gave a rose to Paula to remind her to open herself to the birth of her baby. It just seemed sensible to do, and flowers are often given in love and friendship. In giving this flower, I was not thinking that I was tapping into knowledge which is known and used in other cultures. Symbolic knowledge is as important, or more important, than physical knowledge in the majority of traditional societies. Sexual imagery, stimulative imagery, and religious imagery operate according to symbolic meanings and associations of the objects involved, rather than to the actual physical attributes as perceived in an everyday sense (Bates and Turner 1985: 30). The flower is the symbol of opening. Thus it is not the flower in itself that is important in this sense, but it is the knowledge which understands the flower's symbolic "opening" that gives it its power. Old wives' tales with their spells and remedies, for years discounted as unreliable, were not all harmful and may have contributed to useful traditional childbirth knowledge care by the women healers and midwives (Chamberlain 1981).

Many women have directed their efforts in returning the childbirth experience to women through techniques of mind-body integration (Peterson 1981; Panuthos 1984) or tapping into spiritual energies (Gaskin 1977; Lang 1985). Kitzinger, an internationally known childbirth educator and activist, was one of the first to question techniques which advocated distraction as a means of coping with labor pains. She suggests that these techniques turn women away from the happening in their own bodies. Although many women have used distraction to raise their pain threshold, Kitzinger (1978) encouraged full body awareness (both sensual and sexual) in order to feel the "intense and thrilling sensations" as the vagina opens to birth the baby.

Childbirth education classes sprang up to deliver these promises of a "good birth." Because of the fear of the unknowns of birth, attempts have been made to structure the experience with these many methods. The International Childbirth Education Association and the American Society for Psychoprophylaxis in Obstetrics are two groups that have developed and extended methodological approaches. As well, they are advocates for change in childbirth practices. Over the years there has been increasing recognition that there are strong links between the women's health movement and childbirth organizations. "Both groups attempt to change existing health services; both create alternatives to provide care consistent with their ideals; and both use the process of consciousness raising to increase self-esteem and confidence" (Edwards and Waldorf 1984: 193–94).

Problems. Yet, while there is value in these techniques which have helped many women to prepare for and experience a wonderful and satisfying birth experience, there are problems, too. There is danger of a dogmatism in supposing that there is a "right" way to birth. Although a particular method gives tools for women to use to control their own experience, they sometimes do not work in spite of careful preparation. Those women who lose their own sense of control and experience pain, forceps, drugs, cesarean birth, or long and difficult labors often feel guilty that they have not managed well, or angry that they have not been well prepared. They are left feeling unsure of themselves and their abilities. It may well be that some of the tools of childbirth preparation, such as the breathing patterns and relaxation techniques, come to be used in a technological way, almost like machines. Kitzinger recently described the Lamaze method as "an athletic, goal-oriented blueprint" which basically accepts the male domination of birth (Odent 1984a: xviii).

"If we are to be entirely truthful," said Elizabeth Noble (quoted in CBC 1983: 19), a well-known childbirth educator, "we have to agree that birth is a journey into the unknown, and every couple has to wing it with courage and insight." Even words like "positive," "assertive," and "normal," convey the idea that there is a way to give birth that experts know about. Women, therefore, are faced with their own experience plus a formula which has been set by people who obviously know more than they do. Even if experts have general knowledge about birth, they know very little about a particular birth. Each woman must birth in her own style and uniqueness with support from those who can help her in whichever way is best for her (which may, in fact, include medications and medical intervention).

There is a problem, too, of who controls the educational programs and pays the childbirth educator. Some childbirth educators work within the hospital setting where their allegiance is to a particular hospital and the practices therein. Others feel that the educator should show allegiance solely to her students (expectant parents), and that no institution or doctor should have control over the course content either directly or indirectly (Goer and Euzent 1984: 109). The childbirth educator's dilemma is made even more difficult because of the need to prepare a woman for the reality of obstetrical childbirth and at the same time help her to see beyond its limitations to recognize her own abilities to give birth as she wishes. Yet, the individual woman's childbirth experience should never become the battleground where forms of knowledge are being questioned (Jiménez 1984).

The pragmatic attitude of the various methodologies is especially effective for women who have the economic, intellectual, and social opportunities to take part in childbirth educational programs and to make educated choices about their individual situations. What happens to those who do not have these advantages? Of even more concern is the fact that in the very opportunity of choice there is the possibility that one loses what is of real value. Is what happens in childbirth just a matter of individual choice, with the idea that "what is good for me may not be good for you?" One childbirth educator said, "It is not my goal for all my students to define a safe, satisfying birth experience in the same way I do" (Shearer, B. 1984: 175). Does this mean it is all relative? Should it be a matter for each mother to take responsibility for her own birth, for her own health and the health of her baby? This notion deposits the responsibility of the "good" into the hands of each individual who is situated in a world of diverse forms of knowledge and opinion, in a world of the best salesperson, the best educator, the world of the powerful opinion.

The Critical View

Strengths. The story was told of an obstetrician's reply to a father's request to have other children attend a hospital birth, "Why would you want to have your children see a dirty thing like that?"[1] It is casual remarks like this that demonstrate the need to look at the deep-rooted factors from which such remarks spring. According to Harrison (1982), a doctor herself, many women have experienced the brunt of doctors' attitudes in silence. This silence is being broken through the fluency and clarity of feminist scholars (O'Brien 1981; Oakley 1980b, 1984; Rich 1976; Kitzinger 1962, 1979b, 1983; Morgan 1984).

O'Brien, in stating that human reproduction is inseparable from human consciousness, claims that there can be no analysis from the standpoint of existing theory because the theories themselves are products of male-stream thought (1981: 23). What is needed is to "turn to the fundamental process in which the reproductive relations are grounded and subject it to analysis from a female perspective . . . and from a method of inquiry from which such theory can emerge" (p. 24). The fact that women now have a choice of mothering, that reproduction can be voluntary rather than involuntary, makes it necessary to search for greater understanding of how the process of reproduction influences women's understanding of themselves and the development of knowledge that ensues. It is possible, according to O'Brien, that male reproductive consciousness (alienation through the separation of man from nature and from continuous time) is the basis for the dualistic preoccupation of male philosophy which sees a separation between mind and body, subject and object, past and present, and even, perhaps, male and female (p. 34). She said, "Men have brought to obstetrics the sense of their own alienated parental experience of reproduction and translated it into forms of an objective science" (p. 46). Women mediate their alienation through the act of labor while men appropriate their alienation through objectification and control (p. 32).

The struggle of the critical approach to childbirth knowledge from a feminist perspective strives to uncover the female reproductive consciousness. The male-dominated culture has not given a high value to the creative power of reproductive labor and the act of giving birth (O'Brien 1981: 149). The mediative value of labor *itself* should be brought under scrutiny. The fact that children are born from the labor of women is often ignored, their labor has become something that needs to be "gotten through" in the fastest and easiest way possible. The rapid rise in the cesarean section rate has not been questioned from the point of view that women's active participation in the birth of the child is itself important to the development of the female reproductive consciousness. O'Brien states that women's labor confirms two important issues. "One, obviously, is the knowledge of this child in a concrete sense as *her* child, the product of her labor, a value that her labor has created.

The second is the experience of an integration with the actual continuity of her species" (1981: 151). Paternity, on the other hand, "is essentially an idea—fundamentally abstract, passive," and this problem of the uncertainty of paternity has resulted in the universal oppression of women (1981: 152). The value of labor needs to be reconsidered from the view that it is important for women's own self-understanding, and as an important contribution to society as well. Such reconsideration would acknowledge that women's need to experience childbirth is not a selfish need but one with larger than individual consequences.

O'Brien (1981) and Rothman (1982, 1983) argued that there needs to be a reassessment of the linear view which describes the stages of labor in a rather mechanistic progressive way. The fragmented, unilinear view propagated by obstetrical knowledge and its carriers (the doctor, the hospital, and even prenatal information classes), sweep women into a chronology of pregnancy and childbirth that dissects the experience into logically apprehended, definable, and recognizable events, such as the 40–week pregnancy, or the 12–hour labor. Women now talk of "being late"(Kelpin and Martel 1984).[2] Lateness becomes a concern only when it is contrasted to "being on time," meaning giving birth on the right date. The due date appears to be so important that pregnant women are frequently exposed to ultrasound examination in order to attempt to pinpoint the exact date. Of course, there are considerations which support the desire to know the expected date such as the need to know that the baby is growing adequately and so plans can be made accordingly. But the words "lateness" and "due date" indicate a view that nature should be punctual, that it should know the Gregorian calendar. Without modern obstetrics, women would be less concerned with "lateness." The use of "moments" or cyclical time is more in touch with a woman's natural experience of time, her biological relation to human reproduction. The male experience of discontinuous time (O'Brien 1981: 32) may have precipitated the notion of "time as enemy" to be dominated, controlled, and abstracted. Of course, this is a broad problem related to a concern that with technological control we become less sensitive to the extent to which other things have their own time as well.

Susan Griffin's *Women and Nature* (1978) and *Pornography and Silence* (1981) touch women's realization of their oneness with nature. The objective view of women's bodies, whether finding them "dirty" or "beautiful," or as "machines" to be dominated and managed is a function of the pornographic mind (Griffin 1981). Griffin makes it clear that woman's relationship to nature through her body is a powerful force for integration—integration in body and soul, in mind and emotion—and separation of womb from body as in medical childbirth is cause for the feeling of self-alienation or disintegration. In a society which demands objectivity, which separates nature from culture, which separates body knowledge from language, which sees nature as something to be controlled, there is danger of losing the self.

Consciousness and meaning are part of nature. . . . When bodily knowledge and language are separated, we ourselves experience a terrible separation which ranges all the way from grief to despair to madness. . . . In this way culture destroys a woman's conscious knowledge of her own experience. Just as she is separated from other women, and from her body and her feelings, she is, finally, a stranger to herself. (Griffin 1981: 228, 247)

It is little wonder that women have been willing to accept the domination of scientific obstetrics as, over time, they have been separated and alienated from their own experience. Griffin and others have inspired women to recognize (from Latin *recognōscere*, "to know again") their unity, their oneness with nature and their bodies. In coming to this awareness, women have begun to believe their own strengths to give birth to their own children and are taking back that right.

The impact of technology on childbirth is all-encompassing and pervasive. Franklin (1985) is concerned that women take an active part in changing or developing technology that is fashioned into "a web of life that is intrinsically human." In so doing there may be a way to use technology in a human way rather than to "humanize" it with cosmetic overlays. The values and attitudes of the technological world vary substantially from values of the woman's world. Technology's emphasis on narrow specialization that allows interchange between people and devices, complex hierarchical structures that demand careful planning and scheduling, efficiency and productivity that necessitates the doing of something that is measurable, clash with women's world values. Women, according to Franklin, tend to value flexibility and unpredictability, non-specificity and integration, horizontal structuring with irreplaceable and diverse skills, inventiveness and spontaneity, with emphasis on the ability to cope with a variety of circumstances rather than productivity. Franklin recommended that effort must be made to integrate the values of women's world within the technological order. Women cannot turn away from technology but need to understand its nature (in the struggle for clarity) and to strengthen the bond among women to protect their values (in the struggle for community).

Philosophers (Heidegger 1977a, 1977b; Idhe 1979, 1983; Burch, 1984) suggested that deeper questions need to be asked about the way we live as humans in an environment of technological rationality. In order to question technology one has to step out of the technological frame of reference to explore our relations with machines. Technology is neither neutral nor a mere tool which helps to get the job done. Technology opens up ways of doing things not otherwise possible and this fact means that it also closes down or reduces other possibilities. Burch said that through philosophical reflection we must make an effort to "make ourselves aware of the ways in which technology . . . transforms our experience, [and] limits our perception and understanding," to free us from "the essentially non-technological hold that technology has had upon us." This would make us "free to open ourselves to the fuller range of human possibilities within a relation to technology, possibilities then for putting technology in its place" (1984: 14–15).

Illich, an outspoken critic of modern medicine (1976) and professionalization (1981), said that the existence of "hospitals that spew out the newborn and reabsorb the dying" is a vicious attempt by professionals to replace the nests and snake pits of culture by the sterile wards of professional service (1981: 20). The move to professionalization and its limiting of specialized knowledge to the experts creates needs which then must be met through marketplace practices. The need for expert knowledge and care (the sterile wards) has replaced the common sense knowledge, which in our case is the innate ability of women to birth children within a supportive community (which includes nests and snake pits). There is, of course, value in reducing the trauma of "snake pits," mortality and morbidity, while keeping open the protective "nests" of culture, the support of community.

The marketplace model of childbirth turns childbearing women into consumers or customers, and doctors and other professionals into entrepreneurs or business people. Such a relationship changes care into profit, informed consent into sales contracts, and sees medical research and practice as a thriving business. The business of health care, whose profits make up ten percent of the gross national product in the United States, includes the medical professionals, the manufacturers of costly machinery, the drug companies, the insurance companies, and the government (Edwards and Waldorf 1984: 191). It has also been found that "obstetrician-owned antepartum fetal monitoring equipment is often 'marketed' to pregnant women during prenatal office visits despite four randomized trials which failed to show benefit from these procedures" (M. Shearer 1984: 213). Those who see the market model as important say that the managerial process could result in a carefully formulated program that would allow the doctor to practice medicine and serve the community more effectively and efficiently (Chez 1985). The marketplace model of childbirth becomes one in which the woman is subject to the rationalization of efficiency, expediency, and covering every conceivable risk as criteria from which to judge the procedures. Does this not leave the woman at the mercy of the best salesperson?

Problems. Yet it is possible that these critiques are highly idealistic and removed from the lives of people. Writers like Illich who recommend a return to subsistence living do so with the help of high tech media, communications, and transportation. Are the critics, perhaps, so captivated by their own messages that they fail to see what is right and good in individual circumstances, such as how a woman acts in a world dominated by a powerful form of knowledge that rationalizes itself? Do not these critics of professionalized, sexist, technological, and marketplace childbirth leave women angry and confused, yet impotent to do anything about their individual situations?

Does it not result in antagonism, mistrust, refusal to cooperate, and revolutionary activities which would not have occurred if these scholars did not "stir things up." There is a need to get beyond words and ideas.

It is often suggested that a female doctor, or the increasing number of female doctors in obstetrics, is a turn for the better. This is not necessarily the case. It is understandable that women who have been immersed in the medical approach to childbirth, often working harder than their male counterparts, are not easily critical of their new milieu. Like immigrants, they may tend to seek conformity in language and habit, absorbing the new culture and even defending its system (Franklin 1985). This conformity frequently necessitates compromising their own female experience and results in the breaking of ties with their natural community. Women who do try to maintain these ties with the truth of their own roots often leave their medical practices, or find their place in alternative approaches because personal discrepancies and concessions are too great (Harrison 1982).

Is it not dangerous to suggest, as O'Brien has done, the need to see reproductive labor as valuable or necessary? Would not such an idea support the beliefs by some religious sects and philosophies that women should expect to suffer pain in childbirth? Even Griffin's emphasis on women's ties with nature could be used against women. A return to nature, in any romantic way, would leave women more vulnerable and at the mercy of nature's inequities and catastrophes. Women also are part of the culture that looks at pain as unnecessary and to be avoided, and most would want it to remain that way. We live in a technological world which provides opportunities for control in the most efficient and effective way. While we do not want to deny the value of the instrumental power of technology, we must take care not to be caught in the hegemony of instrumental reasoning.

SELF-UNDERSTANDING

From the above analysis it may appear that forms of knowledge are tied to a particular professional. It may seem, for example, that the doctor, the obstetrician, and the nurse are representative of medical and technological knowledge, midwives and many nurses of midwifery knowledge, birth educators and advocates of methods, and the scholars and/or feminists, of the critical view. Of course, things are not that simplistic. The doctor may use midwifery knowledge from a feminist view. The midwife may be practicing in a hospital that is geared to the pathological situation and be the proponent of obstetrical knowledge. The birth educator may resist marketplace practices and be only interested in preparing individuals for their particular experience with little thought of money. Similarly, the scholar may never have been close to an actual birth, or may, conversely, *be* a nurse, educator, or obstetrician.

If the application of knowledge is related to self-understanding, is there a form of knowledge that can be applied in all situations? Or is there, as has been suggested, one form of knowledge that is appropriate for the high-risk woman, and another for the low-risk woman? Is it only sometimes appropriate, depending on the individual choice, that care is taken so that the environment into which the new baby arrives is one of gentleness, concerned with human touch, concerned with the touch of the family? Is it appropriate for only some women to have access to the fetal monitor or to have a care giver who offers continual support and understanding? Is it appropriate only for women who question the need for drugs and episiotomies to be given the support and time to avoid both?

Meno asked Socrates, the midwife of knowledge, whether virtue is acquired by teaching or by practice or by another way (Sesonske and Fleming 1965). Socrates circumvents Meno's question by asking another question, the question of virtue itself. How often do health care professionals, like Meno, get caught in the question of "how" rather than searching to a deeper meaning of "what" it means to a woman to birth a child? In the childbirth situation nurses, midwives, childbirth educators, yes, even doctors, stand close to the woman in her act of giving birth.[3] Their knowledge, attitude, and care can make the difference by assisting, or opposing women as they come to understand themselves.

It is not necessarily true that one way of approaching birth is more "natural" than another. For many years midwifery knowledge was used exclusively for childbirth. It was the natural way. Now obstetrical knowledge has taken its place. It is now common place. Many breathing patterns taught by various methodologies are not natural, and it not natural to think that labor and its pain has any value for women. It is important to question how the different constructs (knowledge forms) either empower women, or decrease their power to structure childbearing around their own needs and those with whom they live (Hubbard 1984: 332). Each approach to knowledge offers the woman a way to come to grips with her own situation. The way a woman approaches childbirth, that is, which forms of knowledge she encounters, affects how she comes to understand herself. What does a woman learn about herself through her encounter with the application of various forms of childbirth knowledge? In the course of everyday living, the idea of "knowledge forms" does not mean much. The next section explores the possible consequences of a woman's, *Our Woman's*, interaction with approaches to knowledge.

VARIETIES OF WOMEN'S EXPERIENCE

Entering the office to a room full of sick or well people, Our Woman gives her name to the receptionist who retrieves her patient chart. During the initial waiting she stands on the scale, has her blood pressure taken, her urine analyzed, plus any other tests, which are then recorded in clinical numbers on the chart that the nurse retains. After what sometimes seems like an endless wait, Our Woman is escorted to an inner clinical room for another indefinite time. Her chart is put on the outside of the door. This wait gives her time to recall what she may have wanted to ask the doctor once he/she gets there. She reads the doctor's certificates on the wall. Our Woman may investigate the calendar that has interesting drug information, or if she is prepared for this wait, she may read the book or magazine that she has brought for this purpose. The nurse comes in. She may be asked to remove some of her clothes, perhaps from the waist down, and cover herself with the sheet or gown. Most often when the doctor does come in, he/she will read the chart and do whatever further examinations are necessary. There is a moment or two for questions. But Our Woman no longer has any questions. The ones she had are no longer important. After all, the doctor is a busy person with all those others waiting their turn. Anyway, it doesn't matter, because everything seems to be okay. She has passed the inspection for another week or two. Perhaps she will remember her concerns the next time.

Who is this woman? She may be comforted by the authority and protection of obstetrical knowledge experienced throughout her pregnancy and birth. The authority of obstetrical expertise makes it easy for her to say, like Brenda, "Whatever will be will be!" "There is not much I can do about it!" and be grateful for the technology and expertise which give good chances for the birth of a healthy child. She may expect to be looked after, and although she may balk at the patriarchal manner of some doctors who say, "Don't you worry about a thing, my dear, we will look after you," she is trusting of the power of knowledge that makes it possible for anyone to say that. She may see herself as powerless in this situation where independence and self-affirmation are withheld from her. After all, "they" know best. She may even go back to what she may describe as a negative situation a second time. "It is the devil they know," suggested Anna (A2), "At least they know what to expect."

Our Woman's encounter with midwifery knowledge may go something like this. In her visit to the clinic, Our Woman is encouraged to weigh herself, to check her own urine, and to record these measures on her own chart which she carries with her. She waits her turn in a waiting room filled with other pregnant women and babies, for this is the day set aside for women and babies. Over the weeks she develops friendships with others like herself. The midwife or doctor discusses any of the questions and concerns that Our Woman has in an of atmosphere mutual sharing. Perhaps, they talk about who will be attending the birth to look after the other children, or they will go over the diet record that Our Woman has maintained for a week. If she already has children, they may be included in the visit, perhaps even for the physical examination. The midwife also visits the home to discuss preparations for the birth—the supplies needed, suggestions for whom and when to call. Questions that Our Woman may not have brought to the clinic may be discussed more easily in this home setting.

Our Woman, to have access and to choose this alternative approach, has to know that it is available. She is probably like Katherine who said, "I've read a lot about childbirth, and I searched for a place where I could birth my child the way I want. I'm not one to like a lot of intervention in my life." By her very questioning, Our Woman stands against the status quo, the currently accepted practice. She stands determined to make decisions for herself in consultation with those she chooses as childbirth attendants. So for women to request the use of birthing rooms, birth center or home birth, limited intervention, and so on, they must first have the information about the alternative and then must negotiate these privileges which are meted out for the right weight gain, the right laboratory tests, the right dilatation, the right progression and timing, or the right parity. Those women who are not aware of the alternatives or deviate from these "right" attributes automatically receive the benefits and the risks of obstetrical knowledge without question.

The "how-to" methods have offered Our Woman a sense of control of her own situation which she may find helpful and personally strengthening. A particular method will give her something to do, a way to act. But if control is lost, for whatever reason—situational, physical, or emotional— Our Woman senses regret and loss. Loss of control may mean loss of confidence, feelings of guilt, and defeat. The need to control puts Our Woman in an adversarial position of standing up for her rights, being firm, arming herself with her Birth Plan and the latest scientific facts to allow her to maintain that control—at the same time as being in a more vulnerable position with the presence of the child within her body.

What about the self-understanding of Our Woman, the feminist, or Our Woman, who is influenced by technological, professional, and marketplace critiques? She may see herself questioning the domination of certain points of view and see herself fighting for something deeper than her own particular situation. She may feel angry and negative about what she sees as restrictive, oppressive practices while being convinced that childbirth is a time in which she should be able to express herself in a highly intense and personal way. Here Our Woman is left to struggle to find her own way in a world that may not even understand or appreciate her very female nature. She may describe herself as rebellious, like Anna, who said, "It's us against the world."

Yet how does Our Woman, like Jane and Christine, find a physician who is able to work with the nature of women, who does not see women's bodies as machines to be manipulated and controlled in the most efficient way possible? How does she find someone who will not accelerate or slow down her contractions to fit into a linear understanding of labor or the marketplace timetable? How does she find a physician who is not threatened by her demands for equal participation in the decisions surrounding her baby's birth? When or if she does find a doctor who suits her needs, how can she, like Susan, be sure that she will not be transferred to an unknown colleague when nature starts the course of labor in its own time? For many women the support from childbirth groups such as Safe Alternatives in Childbirth, International Childbirth Education Association, or La Leche League, is invaluable. Others choose the support of smaller less organized groups where they, in an atmosphere of trust and friendship, come together with other women to discuss issues central to women's health.

At the present time obstetrical knowledge is so firmly grounded as the appropriate approach that the other forms identified here are the "alternatives." So it is against this environment that women come to deal with themselves and their own situation. They may accept and go with the status quo. They may be subversive and plan a home birth with whatever support is available, for example with midwives in attendance. They may become advocates for better care within the system, like those who make efforts to humanize existing practices. They may become mobile within and use everything to their own advantage. They may be like gadflies and try to deflate the current hegemony.

Our Woman has a choice. In fact, the matter of informed choice is a current obstetrical concern. To make an informed choice means that Our Woman needs to be shown all sides of the picture, the benefits and risks of each option. These opinions may, however, be so entrenched in the particular form of knowledge that there is danger that opinion, itself, is understood as the truth. What is more problematic is that Our Woman may have lost the realization that there is any real choice at all, when for most of her life she has deferred to the experts for basic decisions. Or she may have been trapped by inexorable circumstances where there are few choices. Or, in fact, Our Woman may not even see herself as a person who can choose.

It is Our Woman herself who bears the child that is created hopefully in the act of love within an intimate relationship. Certainly, it is recognized that many women carry and bear children alone, that is, without the support or interest of their partner in the act of conception. Certainly too, many men are actively involved in the coming of the child, so much so, that they can talk of their own internal experience of becoming a father. But, because of women's corporeality, childbearing remains her responsibility and opportunity. In recognizing that giving birth is a personal process for women, we come to see that the birth of the baby is the woman's birth, that is, her birth into motherhood, in close relationship with the child's father. Yet, even the father's view of the birth is externally mediated, and is, in some sense, like that of the doctor, the nurse, the birth educator, and even the courts. For Our Woman to birth a child is indeed to birth herself as a mother, and from those moments to live in the world as a mother.

Chapter 9

Red is the Color of Birth

T here is one moment, within the transformative moments of becoming mother, that gets special attention. It is *that* moment, *the* moment, the *moment of birth*. The moment of birth, this interval, will be the integrative focus of this chapter.

Elsa's Birth[1]

Elsa was born under the full moon / on the first of Spring. / Everyone in the room bore her forth. / My job was in a way the easiest / albeit the most terrifying. / I had to look the Birthforce in the eye / and get out of the way / while it drove through my body / like thunder through tissue paper / demanding that I open up / although with every additional opening / it grew more relentless. . . .

The pain did not lodge in my body / but went out each time, with the note. / There was no wasted energy. . . .

Some time near the end / I pushed / and pushed until I thought my body would break. / The head was out / I heard voices telling me so / but the vibration in the room was mounting strangely / and I could only concentrate harder then ever to meet it. / Finally: expulsion / On hands and knees I felt myself empty. / The relief was stunning. . . .

The room was abuzz with white fear now / but I was not afraid / for Death was in the room, / and in this presence / being afraid would be just plain silly. . . .

So I just looked at the creature in the midwife's arms, no / "positive thoughts," nor "prayers," / just pouring out my soul to that creature / And she gurgled . . . she caught her breath . . . she lived, / soon radiating strength, energy from the love directed / towards her from us and from the universe / that brought her here. I always believed in miracles / but I never thought I'd ever open the door to one. / Everyone who witnessed that door opening was transformed, / because the prize for looking Death in the eye / is Rebirth.

—Jessica Murray, 1983

These excerpts are from one anecdotal image of *the moment of birth*. Strongly felt in Elsa's birth—in all births that I have been a part of—is the tension, the excitement, the fear—"the holding one's breath." We may not call it the "birthforce" but we know what it is when we feel it. It is tied to the wonder of birth and death. It is tied to the spiritual quality of human life. This awesome, mysterious, spiritual dimension of human birth does not mystify women's material experience nor denigrate it. It rather embodies the actual maternal blood and pain in the relationship to the child. When one talks of mystery or the spiritual, it may be easy to think in the abstract as if the spiritual is, in actuality, separate from the concrete reality of physical labor. This dualism leads to the possibility of ignoring the physical reality, minimizing it, negating it, removing it, and subsequently claiming it, as did Christine's doctor.

But "red is the color of birth, bright color of intense joy and severe pain"[2]— a color that forces the questions, "Is the baby okay?" "Will the baby be all right?" as well as the questions "How is the mother?" "How was the labor?" "How was the pain?" It is the momentary stillness—the attentiveness to the first sound, the first breath, or the first cry of the child as an independent being. It is also the recognition of the courage and the love of the woman who gave herself as mother to the moment of birth. It is a respect for the sacredness of the moment that brings a distinct individuality to the child and the mother.

The birth is experienced in some time, some minutes, or some hours. The importance of that actual time is thought to have various interpretations. The birth is experienced through the rhythm of the woman's body, a rhythm of its own, with contractions that come and go, become stronger and longer, and in a sense, take over. The birth is experienced through the social reality of the baby, the heartbeat, the visible head, the smooth, slippery, vernix-covered body, the cry, the look. The birth is experienced by the mother, by the father, and others who support the mother and who greet the child with love, with open arms, and with searching eyes.

Elsa's birth could have taken place anywhere, in a home, or in a hospital, yet in this account the impact of obstetrical, technological knowledge is not strongly felt. But, as obstetrical knowledge is the foundation of birthing practice, perhaps this mother's account is but a fantasy. Does the real picture of birth look more like this?

> A pregnant woman wired up to a machine, electrodes coming out of her every which way so that she looked like a broken robot, an intravenous drip feeding into her arm. Some man with a searchlight looking up between her legs, where she had been shaved, a mere beardless girl, a trayful of bright sterilized knives, everyone with masks on. A co-operative patient. Once they drugged women, induced labor, cut them open, sewed them up. (Atwood 1985: 124)

However, this portrayal may also be merely a caricature.

The impulse behind this work has been to contribute to the development of a philosophy of birth through the exploration of women's experience—a transformation tied primarily to a woman's relationship to the child she bears. My thesis is that women's transformation to mother is central to the development of a philosophy of birth. The experience of carrying, bearing, birthing, and caring for a child gives women knowledge about themselves that is necessary for a comprehensive understanding of our human reality. This knowledge comes from women's experience; and as we take serious this knowledge, we are helped to make decisions about difficult aspects of human life—abortion, reproductive technologies, appropriate use of technology, appropriate research, the place of birth, and policies and practices surrounding birth.

EAR ON THE BELLY: HOW WE LISTEN

In this section, I will explore the effect of technology on the moment of birth using, as an example, the fetal monitor.

> We used to keep in touch with a baby's heart, its trepidation or distress, by putting our ear close, and listening, listening sometimes even heart to heart. Now, we turn away from the baby. We look at abstractions on a foetal monitor. The practice estranges us, even when we realize theoretically that it does. (Laing 1982: 16)

Tools have been used in childbirth for years. We have listened to the fetal heart, by auscultation, since as early as 1816. In the last years listening to the baby's heartbeat has moved away from the woman's belly, to the end of the stethoscope, to the other side of the room, to another room, and even to another town! According to Tucker (1979: 116–18), displays are developed so that professionals can view a number of patients simultaneously; alarm systems include a computer printout identifying the problem, for example, "Room 3, severe variable deceleration;" and telephone transmission of the fetal monitoring data can be sent from a small rural hospital to a major perinatal center for expert assessment. The monitor also records the frequency, duration, and relative intensity of the woman's contractions, and the resting time between contractions. Such advances in technology are important, yet need careful scrutiny. No longer is the ear on the belly needed to *hear* the fetal heart rate, nor the touch of the hand needed to *feel* the hardness of the uterine wall during the woman's contraction.

Laing claims that the use of the monitor estranges. The dictionary says estrange means "to remove from an accustomed place or association; to put at a distance, especially a psychological distance; or to disrupt a bond that existed between one or more persons; to make (a person) a stranger" (Oxford English Dictionary 1971). How does the use of the fetal monitor estrange? Who is troubled by the estrangement? Is the estrangement important in the larger picture? And even if we understand theoretically what is a risk, will we be able to do anything about it? And would we want to?

Starkman (1977), Shields (1978), Molfese, Sunshine, and Bennett (1982) investigated women's experiences with and reaction to the use of the fetal monitor during their labor. These studies began from a position that the monitor will be used in labor and recommended the need for appropriate information so that women understand its use and accept its application. Of course, if obstetricians have lost their ability to listen to the fetal heartbeat in clinical ways, as reported by Christine, there is no choice.

Listening to the Woman

The rhythm of contractions takes central focus in the moment of birth. I recall them vividly. I remember the beginning, thinking "Oh, here we go again," and the ending—the big breath, the momentary reprieve. As the contractions became more powerful—they took on a life of their own—there was nothing to do but let them pass. With the monitor the contractions can be viewed, or "felt," by others in the room—by the staff and the woman's partner. This visual understanding of the contraction may change the experience of the contraction for the woman. She no longer needs to say to herself and others, "Here we go again," but can be told by others that she is having a contraction. While "it is interesting to watch," said Katherine, "if you start watching it you are not necessarily in touch with what you are feeling" (K3). In losing a sense of what one is feeling, it is easier to be directed by others as Melissa pointed out, "They, the doctor and my husband, could really coach because they could see when the contractions were coming without having to ask a lot of questions of me, or wonder where I was at" (M).

Other women felt that the monitor helped the husband or partner to feel more involved in the labor. The husband/partner may now even seem to know more about the contraction than the woman herself. Christine said, "He felt more involved because he could say [to me], 'That was a strong one' and that would encourage me because I made it through it. He could feed that information to me" (C3). At the same time, though, Christine described very clearly what her own contractions were like.

> I found I had basically two types [of contractions], one that would build very quickly and peak almost immediately, and I could tell if I was going to have one. On the first sign, "Oh, it is going to be another one of those," and I knew it. The others would build much slower and be longer, but they would not be nearly as intense and I could tell when I was going to have one of them too.

So although she says that the monitor was helpful for Nathan to give her information about her contractions, Christine could describe very specifically what her contractions were like herself. Len also described the monitor as invaluable in giving him information about Natasha's contractions. Len said he would have felt helpless if he did not have the monitor to tell when the contractions were starting so he could give directions to Natasha (N). However, Natasha said later, "I wanted to do it on my own and I felt capable, but I don't think that you are altogether there. I was relying more on what Len thought than on what I thought" (N).

Anna did not have access to a fetal monitor. Bill talked about how he worked with Anna, breathing with her with each contraction and stroking her body as she relaxed between the contractions. He said, "I felt so much a part of it." It is possible that the partner's help and involvement is equally or more desirable if he can observe the woman's experience of the contraction with his hand on her abdomen, focusing and sharing his attention with her to attune themselves to the rhythm and nature of her labor as she feels it. While on the surface it may seem that the monitor promotes the working together of the partners through labor, it may, in actuality, incline women to depend more and more on others to give information about themselves. They come to rely less on what they themselves think and experience, which may lead them to be robbed of their self-confidence and the feeling that they could manage for themselves (Dunn 1979).

Some women felt the information displayed on the monitor was all the information that was needed in their care. Yvonne felt that the nurse wanted her just to go to bed with the monitor on, because other information, such as how the contractions were being experienced by the woman, was not as important, or indeed essential. Another woman said that her obstetrician would "know everything that was happening to me just by watching the machine" (Starkman 1977: 501).

The bodily experience of contractions in the moment of birth is changed by the fetal monitor, and this change may affect the way women come to understand their own experience. On the one hand, without the monitor, Victoria could say, "It was an incredible experience—I wouldn't have thought I could be so in touch with my body." On the other hand, towards the end of labor, with the internal monitor in place, Christine had difficulty knowing if and when she was having contractions at all and needed to be told. She said, "I literally could not tell you if this was just my muscles aching from pushing or if this was a contraction. And I said to Nathan, 'You will have to tell me. I cannot feel when it starts' " (C3). Neither could Christine tell that she was ready to birth but learned from the doctor's appearance. "The doctor was getting ready for delivery because I remember him coming out in various stages of green. He was getting more green each time he came in [laughs]." And she talked of being closed. "I felt tight, terribly tight. I felt tight and that nothing was coming to the bottom, nothing [referring to the baby] was coming to where it should be (C3)." Christine had lost a sense of her own contractions, heard and experienced her baby outside herself, and could only tell that she was getting ready for delivery because the doctor was getting dressed in the appropriate clothes. Attached to a fetal monitor, the uterine activity of the woman is displayed with such clarity that it is possible for the readings to become the primary focus of everyone, even Christine. Such a situation may have affected Christine's sense of her own rhythmic contractions and her inner experience of moving her baby out of her body. Thus, we begin to see the danger of technology. According to Blumenfeld, the danger is that it "tends to cultivate insensitivity, a clinical detachment, a deadening of emotions. And nothing is more dangerous to human survival than that, for our emotions are our survival instincts, and when we shut them off we begin to lose our way, to be less human" (1975: 195).

Listening to the Baby

Is the baby okay? With the use of the fetal monitor, this question is partly answered—even before the birth itself. This is powerful and dramatic.

That is where it was, over there! That is where the noise was, where his heart was! There! I could hear it all the time (C3).

Christine had just said, "I didn't think much about the baby and the reason I didn't was because I could hear his heartbeat. I could hear his heart thumping all the time and it was fine" (C3). The baby's vital function, the heartbeat, is heard in the machine.

For many months the childbearing woman has felt the baby through the inner movements, the stretches, the turns, the hiccups; has seen the bumps, the kicks, the ripples across her stomach, has encouraged others—partners, and mothers—to "come and feel." She has listened, in wonder, to the heartbeat through the stethoscope or the Doppler, and counted the beats, guessing on the sex. Attached to the fetal monitor, either with a large strap surrounding her abdomen, or by a wire attached through her cervix to the baby's scalp, the woman now listens to or watches on a screen, her baby's heartbeat as the others do—the doctor and the father. That is, everyone (mother, father, doctor, and others) can now hear and/or see the record of the baby's heartbeat. It is fascinating. These interested observers, sometimes with a mechanic, may hover around the machine. While dramatic, and reassuring of the baby's liveliness, the baby *in the machine* changes the focus of everyone, even the mother.

Wendy found the monitor extremely helpful. "It was just numbers you could see on the monitor," she said, "but I knew that the baby wasn't in any kind of distress, that she was coping well with the contractions" (W). Although Wendy originally did not want to have the fetal monitor attached, she found it reassuring for herself to know that her baby was fine. She did not have to depend on the staff to tell her about the well-being of her baby. While many women may find the monitor interesting and helpful, some experience the baby in the machine as a source of confusion and fright. Melissa said, "It [the monitor] wasn't functioning particularly well either, which was a drawback. It kept going to its emergency BEEP, and it sounded very ominous, and it would go beep and she [the nurse] would come tearing in to see what was wrong. Our reaction was to say that it is something with the monitor, not with the child" (M).

In one sense it would seem that the fetal monitor could support the intertwining presence of the baby within the life of the women, as the heartbeat of the baby and the contractions of the women are, together, so vividly displayed and recorded. One might expect this information could assist women to be "in" the contraction. In another sense the mother/baby unity is disrupted by the recordings—as each stand alone, for everyone to see.

So in spite of the drama of hearing the heartbeat telling the mother, father, and attending staff about the health of the baby there are other, less obvious, things that are also occurring. The experience of hearing the baby "over there" may make it harder for the woman to open herself to push her baby into the world with the strength and intuitive knowing of her own birthing body. Montagu's notion that "the uterine contractions of labor constitute the beginning caressing of the baby in the right way" (1971: 72) may seem strange in thinking of Christine's experience. It would be hard to feel contractions as "internal caresses" of the baby while listening to or experiencing one's baby in a machine. At the same time it needs to be remembered that the fetal heart rate is a first indication of problems needing prompt medical attention which can save the life of the baby. Thus, the fetal monitor is an important tool in listening to the baby and answering the question of the baby's health. It is a matter of how the "listening for the baby" occurs.

REACHING OUT TO THE BABY: HOW WE WELCOME

Then the family stills to view one of the truly astonishing wonders of life: the first breath. As Jonathan takes his first gulp of oxygen, his complexion slowly warms from an eerie blue to a glowing pink. . . . The joy of the family is palpable. They fuss. They adore. They coo. Jonathan responds . . . he is wide-eyed but lies serene in mother's arms. (McRoberts 1984)

This description of the baby's first breath was written by a newspaper reporter who attended a birth. Here is another description of the first breath—by a father. He writes, "Sara was born. . . . We put our hands on her head, we caressed the warm, moist body, and felt her chest expand with the first breath of life, and then heard her let out her first cry" (Personal Communication, Russell Kelly, June, 1987).

But others have described the first breath differently. A respected obstetrician, an advocate for the use of fetal monitors with all laboring women, agrees that the first minutes of the life of a newborn infant *are* most important. "But," he says, "it is not in the dim light in the delivery room [referring here to the Leboyer method] . . . or . . . early skin contact [in reference to the work of Klaus and Kennell] . . . but [it is] warmth, a normal Apgar score, and a high umbilical cord pH which are really important" (Baumgarten 1981: 271). The language displays opposing views of the baby's first breath. The last voice may be said to express an "objective view" and the first two "romantic subjective prattle." But what is the experience of the baby, and the family, in each situation? Can we know?

We live in language; language is a way, a mode of being in the world (Smith 1983)—or according to Heidegger, "Man [*sic*] is language" (Idhe 1983). Words are a testament to our life. What do the words tell us? The language points to the whole context in which the baby takes that first breath and the way the baby is welcomed. In each situation, what is sought is a healthy baby and mother, but we notice that divergent forms of knowledge are used to achieve that outcome. In the views of the reporter and father, we see a welcome encompassing a respect for the wonder of a new life (that independent breath), the response of the family (warm caresses, palpable joy), the response of the baby (change in color, wide-eyed, serene, the first cry) in the arms of the family. In the obstetrician's account, the goal of environmental warmth (possibly a warm blanket, or an incubator), a normal Apgar score (evaluation of the baby's heart rate, respiratory effort, muscle tone, reflex irritability, and color), and a high umbilical cord pH (blood sample taken from the cord) has lost all trace of Jonathan or Sara, or any baby, the mother, the family, and even, perhaps, respect for the wonder of life. What is heard, rather, is measurement and calculation in a vacuum of any human interaction.

The Husserlian understanding of intentionality, that all consciousness is consciousness of "something," helps us to understand. "At its depth, intentionality may be described as the *foundational correlation rule* of phenomenology by which any possible knowledge whatsoever is located and circumscribed" (Ihde 1983: 146). This is shown by the correlation between *noema*, the "what" (object-correlate) that is experienced and *noesis*, the "way" in which that object is experienced (subject-correlate). To understand the experience we need to take account of the what, the outcome, to which that experience is directed. Therefore, if what is seen as most important to experience in the first moments of life is the fixed, quantitative, measurable value of the Apgar score and the cord pH, then the mode of experiencing will tend to be quantitatively, technologically colored, using measures, scales, and machines to reach for that end. Conversely, if what is most important is for Jonathan and Sara to take their first breath in the arms of the parents, then how that comes to be experienced will be more involved with helping the baby take that breath with massage, with caressing hands, with open arms, and with "cooing" encouragement.

Let us now look at another situation where a baby is welcomed. Here are the words of the grandmother who was present at the birth of Anna's second child.

> And then the baby came. And first thing I heard "it's a girl." And we looked and this little girl wouldn't breathe. And I thought to myself, "It's okay, Anna, you can have another one." That went through my mind. I didn't say it, I just felt it. And the next thing I thought, "Don't do that to my daughter. She worked so hard for you, for nine months and worked hours and hours. Don't do that to her." I felt really angry with her—for not breathing and giving Anna such a rough time. I couldn't get rid of that feeling until the next morning when I had a cry on someone's shoulder. . . . It was scary. They massaged baby and moved her legs. And Anna kept saying, "Come on little one, come on little one, come on little one." The heart was always beating and that was a good thing. . . . The critical moment for Alexandra was when the midwives put her on Anna's tummy after she had caught herself, not really rhythmic yet, put her on Anna's tummy and then she got her color and "that was it." (Personal Communication, mother of Anna, February 21, 1987)

It was scary! We can feel the terror, and the anger, in the grandmother's words.

This example, again, shows the difference between meeting the world "in the flesh" (based on knowledge of human relationships, with attributes of encouragement and even anger) or "through machines" (based on knowledge of blood levels and measurement). Both outcomes can be in the interest of the health and safety of the mother and child, but the criteria for reaching toward that safety has to do with the whole context in which the health of the baby is sought and the way in which the baby is welcomed.

The moment of birth as a welcoming, as a community event, seems rather strange when we consider most births in the hospital where only one companion is allowed to accompany the birthing woman. Jane's mother had wanted to be present at Lisa's birth, but even in a birthing room, Jane could have only one person, her husband, with her. Nevertheless, Jane's mother slipped in, unobtrusively, to see her daughter and granddaughter within minutes of the birth (J3). In the hospital at the moment of birth, the mother is generally surrounded by strangers—nurses whose names Christine could not even remember (C3). At home, the grandmother was present as a supporting member of the welcoming community—perhaps even with her anger, as the she herself suggested.

> Sure it was a traumatic and scary moment for all of us, yet we felt we were all a part of giving life to this little one—even if it meant being angry with her. As a matter of fact, talking about it now, I understand the positive part of anger. I didn't before. I felt guilty for being angry.

We take the technological approach, with its community of strangers, for granted. Even the new birthing rooms (the places in which "normal" births take place) are equipped with all the latest technological machines—the fetal monitor, intravenous supplies, suction apparatus, the respirator, scales, test tubes, the incubator—however well they may be hidden behind the colorful curtains, flowery wallpaper, and collapsible oak bed. Of course, the Apgar score is a valued tool, giving important assessment of the baby's function, and the cord pH gives clues about dangerous chemical imbalances. The fetal monitor, too, does give the health care professionals information important to the care of the woman and baby. Yet, we must remind ourselves that these technologies are not neutral; and as we surround ourselves with the "natural" technological influence, we need to take care, to consider how technology mediates the experience for the baby, for the woman, for the community of family and friends, and for the care givers.

With the use of a monitor that could give information that in some ways is more accurate than a woman herself could give, a scenario can be envisioned where the woman need not speak at all. In fact she would have nothing to say because there would no longer be any words to describe her sensation of painful contractions. In such a situation others could direct and control her labor, telling her when her contractions are starting and finishing. She would not experience her baby inside but rather as a separate being who is delivered through the coordinated efforts of others. She would just be the vehicle of the child's passage into the world where he or she will be kept warm, measured, and tested. It would be hard to tell the difference between the woman and the machine because they would all act machine-like with wires and electrodes attaching themselves together. In order to avoid such an extreme caricature, consideration must be given to how women come to communicate with health care professionals, what language is used; how husbands and friends support women in their birthing process; how women are separated from their babies, even before birth; how machines almost seem like humans; and more importantly, how humans come to act like machines.

Appropriate Technology

One of the most difficult concerns, according to the philosopher Robert Burch, is that while technology opens up a whole range of possible experiences, it also narrows our experience in certain ways. The challenge, he said "is to decide how these . . . possibilities can be kept in a *properly human context*" (1984: 14)—a context that seeks to understand the totality of human experience. In order to question technology as it invades aspects of our lives, we must reassess what it means to be human. Once we open ourselves to the question of meaning, and the place of technology in human life, we find that we must make choices, which according to Heidegger (1977b) is the "freeing claim." In this freedom, this choosing, is the envisioning of our human position with regard to things, to machines, even to a machine like the fetal monitor.

Weizenbaum (1976), a professor of computer science who created the computer program ELIZA to play the role of Rogerian psychotherapist, began to question the morality of his actions when he realized the dangers of people yielding "autonomy to a world viewed as machine" (p. 9). He began to see that the power to choose, beyond the calculation of instrumental reasoning, is necessary to stop the erosion of our humanity where a birthing woman and her child are treated as less than whole persons, when "patients are more and more merely passive objects on whom cures are wrought and to whom things are done" (Weizenbaum 1976: 259). Passivity and dehumanization occur when:

> people's own inner healing resources, their capacities for self-reintegration, whether psychic or physical, are more and more regarded as irrelevant in a medicine that can hardly distinguish a human patient from a manufactured object . . . [when a person] no longer even senses himself, his body, directly, but only through pointer readings, flashing lights, and buzzing sounds produced by instruments attached to him as speedometers are attached to automobiles. (Weizenbaum 1976: 259)

The primary health care concept of appropriate use of technology is seen as the impetus to "break the chains of dependence on unproved, oversophisticated, and overcostly health technology" (Mahler 1981: 10). Yet technology, to be appropriate, must not only be technically sound, culturally acceptable, and financially feasible, but must also contain or enlarge the vision of our humanity, a vision that encourages the individual to depend on herself with the support of community, not as a mere actress in a drama written and orchestrated by others. We must never give up the power to make choices, to move beyond technical decision-making or simple problem-solving techniques, if we are to develop and use the burgeoning technology appropriately. These kinds of choices have to be concerned not only with expediency, efficiency and cost-effectiveness but with contextuality, relationship, self-reliance, caring, respect, and courage. The red color of birth, the interaction of joy and pain, the attributes of respect, love, and courage, are not technical issues, and therefore need attention that is not merely tied to technological reasoning and action, or limited to technological solutions.

Appropriate Knowledge

The birthdays of my children are times when I often reminisce with the children and their father about our experience of each moment of birth. We remember the day, when the contractions started, where I was, when I decided to go to the hospital, what they looked like as babies, who was there, and so on. Although we tell their birth stories again and again, each telling is meaningful for me and, I think, interesting and important for them, as well. They are transforming stories: ones that changed my life.

Yet the stories of the moments of birth are not merely individual experiences that many women share. The stories of birth show how women come to understand themselves, and how women come to understand themselves is a larger issue than attention to individual stories would suggest. It has to do with how women come to understand the world, thus influencing the very foundations of forms of knowledge. It may not be incidental that obstetrical knowledge has been tied to male-developed, objective, abstract thought, nor it may not be incidental that midwifery knowledge is tied to women's experience of reproduction—as a normal, contextual, social process of individual and community life. They may indeed reflect the experience of childbirth from two different views leading to the development of different knowledge.

If O'Brien (1981) is right that male reproductive consciousness (becoming fathers) influences men's ability to think in abstract and objective ways, further exploration of women's reproductive consciousness (becoming mothers) will provide forms of knowledge that swerve away from detached analysis to approaches that are tied to concrete experience of relationship and integration. Such approaches to knowledge may avoid the polemic of mind-body, subject-object, natural-technological, masculine-feminine, or obstetrical-midwifery. Knowledge that integrates mind-body, subject-object, nature-technology, may also come to be seen as valuable in learning more about living as humans in this world.

Chapter 10

Living the Questions: One Is What One Does

The transformative experience that is accessible to women who become mothers has been the central focus of this book. The conversations with women have opened ways to explore what it means to become a mother, requiring a questioning of the forms of knowledge used by women to understand themselves as mothers. Being a mother is a matter not only of the mother role (Barber and Skaggs 1975; Wolkind and Zajicek 1981), not only of caring for the child, not only of caring for a home. It *is* a matter of a changed understanding of who women *are* as mothers. Becoming a mother is a matter not only of maternal tasks (Rubin 1984), not only of developmental tasks (Valentine 1982), not only of stressors and satisfactions (Wilson 1982). It is a realization and acceptance that "I *am* a mother."

Of course, no woman's life is exactly alike, as demonstrated by the stories of Brenda, Christine, Jane, Susan, Anna, and Katherine. Each woman is individual, and her appropriation of this phenomenon is unique. The themes, the moments, that emerged from individual life experiences were developed in a dialogical way so as to explore their meanings for other women as well. As I entered into a relationship with the text of the stories, the transcripts (of these six women and many others), literature about childbearing and mothering, other phenomenological literature, and my own experience, the search for understanding of women's experience became broader than the unique meaning of individual lives. Yet the explorations of individual experiences made it possible to see the importance of the broader issues.

The orientation in the approach to the texts has been to search for an understanding of women in a way that acknowledges the public reality of women's private lives. This public/cultural responsibility is realized in the care that pregnant and childbearing women receive and in issues that affect the mothering aspect of women's lives. The hermeneutic thrust of this study has aimed at producing a text that reveals a strong version of women's lives, one that shows the hopes as well as the challenges that childbearing brings. In the attempt to understand by writing, reflection, and re-writing, there is an underlying recognition that the depth of human life may become flattened, simplified, and even polarized, in such an attempt. The goal has been the opposite—to write in a way that reveals the layers of complexity of human life in present society. With women's changing understanding of themselves this revealing has challenged existing notions and explored new ideas.

Exploration of issues of meaning (questioning human values) sometimes may seem to focus on the extremes. Attention to the less traditional, the unusual, could be criticized as a one-sided pointing to the problems of one viewpoint while disregarding the problems inherent in another. On the one hand, in bringing the less dominant approach to childbirth knowledge and experience to light, there is a danger of overstating or simplifying the situation. On the other hand, it is primarily because there has been a dominant, one-sided practice of childbirth that the effort to create a more balanced view (while seeming to be only critical) may be necessary.

As I write this final chapter, I acknowledge that in many ways the question of "How can I understand women's transformation to mother?" is still present. But it can be said that all questions of this nature are, in reality, ongoing. The intimate relationship that exists between questioning and understanding, between showing and hiding, is what gives the hermeneutic experience its true dimension (Gadamer 1975) and makes the project of uncovering the meaning of something difficult. Women's lives are rapidly changing, and will continue to change, as they learn to understand themselves in new ways. So while this text has revealed many aspects of women's lives in tracing their transformation to mothers, essential aspects may remain hidden. Therefore, one needs to remain open to knowing more about this transformative experience. What does it mean to be a mother? Such questions demonstrate the open-endedness, the on-goingness of this research. So, in a sense, it *is* not finished. Indeed, it *cannot* be finished.

Therefore, the questioning goes on in the day-to-day choices one makes, the interests one pursues, and commitments one undertakes. If one agrees with Weizenbaum that "the salvation of the world depends only on the individual whose world it is" (1976: 267), then each individual must first discharge that responsibility in their own life as a responsibility to the larger community. For me, "living the questions" of this book has invited reassessment of my commitment to work in the area of health care, with learning and teaching, with women and children, with technological changes, with birth and death, striving for an attitude of courage. "Living the questions" means reassessing my responsibility for my actions including how I live as a mother to my children. "Living the questions" means that I need to reflect on what I have done within the parameters of this research and my responsibility to the women of the study. Recall the birth of Suzie, Brenda's baby (Chapter 2). Her father and I could have picked her up and welcomed her to this world. The nurse-midwife could have spent those few minutes helping the father reach for the child he watched so attentively. The doctor could have talked to the baby and her parents in ways that would have encouraged a celebration of this important moment. Not one of us did anything. We carried on with our procedures, our charting, and our watching. Everyone felt uncomfortable that Brenda could not reach out to her baby, but we did nothing to assist her. I did nothing, and this knowledge leaves me troubled. Yet in the effort to ask what we must do, we must not forget that the essential concern must be with what we must be. In real life, however, being and doing are not separate aspects of living, for one *is* what one *does*.

To find an example for health care professions I look to Florence Nightingale. Florence Nightingale has been immortalized as "The Lady with the Lamp." Apparently, though, Florence was also called "The Lady with the Hammer," for during the Crimean war in Turkey, "while in charge of the nursing in the military hospitals, she was refused the key to the store-room door. With a hammer, she broke open the door" (Kramarae and Treichler 1985: 23).

Recall the ancient, pre-Christian myth of Eros (Amor, Cupid) and Psyche. The myth, which is a product of the collective imagination and experience, portrays the human condition with indelible accuracy (Johnson 1976). Beautiful Psyche was married to the god of love, Eros. She lived in paradise, happy to be loved by Eros who, although he would not let her see his face, came to sleep with her each night. By listening to her sisters, Psyche became convinced that she needed to see the reality of Eros. She needed to see his face. One night as she took a lamp and lit it, she saw his beauty—"the most beautiful creature in all of Mount Olympus"—and fell in love with him. In her attempt to get near him, Psyche awakened him with hot oil spilled from her lamp. He understood what she had done. He became angry with her. He left her. Psyche, then, had to win back Eros's love through her own work—through various tasks and difficulties.

"The symbol of the lamp in the myth points to the light-bearing capacity of women," said Johnson, "In the Eleusinian mysteries, the women carry torches, which shed a peculiarly feminine kind of light. A torch lights up the immediate surroundings, shows the practical next step to be taken" (1976: 27). The word "lamp" comes from Greek *lampein* meaning "to shine." A simple device, one could say. Yet in its shining the lamp lights the way, shows the next step, lights up the immediate surroundings, reveals the beauty of the situation, stimulates the anger, and leads to action. The lamp associated with Florence and Psyche was a hand-held lamp. In order to show the way the lamp needs to be carried by a person, a nurse, a midwife, or a doctor. A machine will not do. Florence, the lady with the lamp, reminds the care giver to *be* there with a light to show the way, to illuminate the dark space, to provide a circle (of support) in which the woman who becomes mother can do what she needs to do. The lamp reminds one what one must be.

Florence used the hammer in order to do what she needed to do. The hammer is a tool for destruction and building. Nietzsche also talked about the use of the hammer—called his "philosophy of the hammer" (Morgan 1941; Kaufmann 1968). Nietzsche's hammer was "intended to smash what is rotten in humanity and hew out what is sound" (Morgan 1941: 357). Nietzsche was reacting against the "vast social machine in which individuals are equal and trivial parts, [where] everything is means, nothing an end," leading to "safety, comfort, and mediocrity for everybody" which he called a slow stagnation (Morgan: 354). He was striving for a reassessment of all values. He wanted the conscious (those who saw the situation) to become courageous, the silent to become outspoken, in order to bring to illumination the true nature of traditional values (Kaufmann 1968). "Florence with the hammer" reminds the health care professional that it may be necessary to tear down those structures which interfere with personal growth and responsibility, and to destroy that which holds individuals to consider only the expedient rather than the meaningful. The hammer can also be used to build a society, an environment, that is not machine-like, but one that appreciates individual uniqueness and individual projects of living. The hammer reminds one what one must do.

While thoughts of the lamp and the hammer, of being and doing, can be helpful, the project of "living the questions" raised in this book is not easily carried out. It means keeping open the search for understanding, constantly questioning what is taken as secure, accepting that there is still more to learn, searching for another view of the complex reality of living—which may open further depths of questioning and understanding. It means, also, keeping open the conversations among women, between groups of women who tend to polarize women's issues such as particular feminist groups and pro-family groups. It means keeping open conversations among women and men about unique and shared ways they come to their experience of parenting. It means keeping conversation open among nurses, midwives, doctors, researchers, and scholars, to explore forms of knowledge which enlarge our humanity rather than narrow it. It means keeping open conversations with the professionals, technicians, and the marketplace entrepreneurs, to avoid attachments to knowledge for technical, sexist, or economic reasons. It means keeping open questions of how women live as mothers in dialogue with questions of the place of children in society. It means developing community. "Living the questions" is an ongoing project.

Such conversations are needed to discuss the significance, the possibility, and the consequences of differing approaches to childbirth knowledge in order to change attitude and practice. This is not the place to advocate solutions to the problems raised in this work. Simplistic solutions will not do. I hope, however, that this study may help in the process of clarifying the social and medical issues, the personal meanings, and the taken-for-granted childbirth practices needed to produce productive dialogue. In the following section of this chapter I present conclusions derived from the present study that are necessary suppositions for the continuation of dialogue about knowledge used in childbirth education and practice.

CONCLUSIONS

Giving birth to a child is a transformative experience for women.

Policies regarding childbirth practices need to include the recognition that childbirth is a transforming experience for women. Planning for the health and safety of the mother and child needs to include recognition of the woman's own experience of becoming a mother.

The woman is changed by the experience of bearing a child. She is not a mere vessel, but is an active, growing, changing participant.

The decision to become a mother is more complex than the rational decision-making process can encompass.

To make a decision to bring a child into one's life is to enter into change that one cannot really comprehend. The decision to have a child is beyond mere problem-solving.

Having a home for a child, is to take on a new responsibility for the world—the world as a good place for children.

Childbirth is a sexual experience, not just at conception but throughout pregnancy, birth, and nourishment of a child.

Deciding to accept a child into one's life is an ongoing decision. It must be re-affirmed at various times in the growth of both mother and child.

The intertwining presence of the child in a woman's body needs to be held sacred at all times during pregnancy and birth so that the woman can experience her own change through this unique relationship.

The process of becoming a mother for a woman who adopts, fosters, or hires a surrogate, may be different than for a woman who "carries the child beneath her heart." Exploring different experiences may show the significance of each in a clearer light.

The pregnant woman is changed by the presence of the child. While maintaining all her own projects of living, the pregnant woman is also growing with her developing baby. It is a healthy, unique, bodily experience.

Maternity clothes need to support a woman's move to mother—helping her to accept and feel good about her growing body as a sexual and powerful being.

The vulnerability that a woman begins to feel in pregnancy is not a sign of weakness but a sign of the increasing need for her relationship with others. A woman "with child" is a community responsibility.

The time-table approach to pregnancy and birth denies the individual variations in this developmental process. Care needs to be taken to ensure that normal, individual variations are not seen as pathological.

A woman "with child" experiences a changed approach to the world. Becoming a mother begins with this changed view of the world.

The separation of the mother and child through labor and its pain offer the possibility of integration and wholeness for both woman and child.

Pain is not always negative. It can be healthy, and lead to personal growth. Childbirth pain cannot be compared to the pain of illness. It is different. It produces a child.

Women need support to deal with their pain through a number of ways, finding a good position, making noise, being themselves, having familiar people and things, breathing patterns, as well as medication. Support should be given, without asking, in all birth environments—hospitals, birthing rooms, birthing centers, or home.

The rhythm of labor can be useful in helping women deal with their pain. Learning to get in touch with their own bodily rhythm can prepare women for labor.

The place of birth, be it hospital, birthing room, birth center, home— needs to be an environment where the fullness and richness of the moment of birth can be experienced. The mother (with child) needs central prominence in the place of birth: the care givers need to be cooperative.

"Being in pain" is an inner process of women that must be respected and supported.

The separation that occurs in childbirth makes possible the wholeness of both mother and child. Separation is not a negative process, but a necessary occurrence that is gradual and, probably, never complete.

The experience of childbirth may bring women closer to other women, as well as to partners and friends, who are a part of this sacred human experience.

The responsibility of becoming a mother belongs to women. All procedures, techniques, and interventions, to the woman or child, need to consider and support the acceptance of responsibility on the part of the mother. Responsibility must never be usurped by others.

Responsibility for the life of the child contains the possibility and impact of death.

Giving birth is women's responsibility. Taking that responsibility is an opportunity for growth. Labor is a necessary and valuable experience for women. If women are not able to "give" birth, they need to have the opportunity to reflect on their own experiences with those who assisted with the birth.

Preparing to take responsibility affects the moment of birth.

As a part of her sexual nature, childbirth for women should be seen as the opportunity for fulfillment and satisfaction.

To be responsible for the world begins with the recognition that women's experiences may not be fully valued and respected.

To be responsible for the world includes attitudes that will empower a girl/woman rather than restrict her.

To have a child on one's mind is to be a mother. Support for women who are mothers is needed so they can care for their children in the best way possible—through shared parenting with the child's father or other caring adults, supportive child care arrangements, flexible work hours, shared job opportunities, etc. Women need support to mother their children.

To have a child in one's life is a blessing.

To have a child in one's life forces one to think about how one should live.

To have a child in one's life means one no longer is able to live only for oneself.

This particular exploration of women's experience of becoming a parent brings to light the need to explore men's experience. Parenting is a shared undertaking—parenting by both mothers and fathers is needed by children.

NOTES

Chapter 1

1. This book is based on conversations with many women. Data from the conversations with the six women who provided the primary source of information are Anna (A1–7)—seven interviews between October 15, 1984 and June 1, 1986; Brenda (B1–6)—six interviews between October 28, 1984 and November 1, 1985; Christine (C1–8)—eight interviews between February 17, 1984 and June 8, 1986; Jane (J1–6)— six interviews between February 16, 1984 and October 16, 1985; Katherine (1–6)— six interviews between September 17, 1984 and June 15, 1986; and Susan (S1–7)— seven interviews between October 15, 1984 and June 16, 1986. Women interviewed for an earlier version of Chapter 5 during January and February, 1983 were Diane (D), Ellie (E), Flo (F), Helen (H), Iris (I), Laura (L), Noa (N), Victoria (V), and Xavier (X). Women interviewed for an earlier version of Chapter 9 during December 1984 were Melissa (M), Natasha (N), Opal (O), Una (U), Wendy (W), and Yvonne (Y). Other women quoted here include Gail (G), August 8, 1986; Paula (P1–3), May 7–10, 1983 and January 6, 1986. All names have been changed to preserve anonymity.
2. This policy varied from hospital to hospital, and from community to community. In some places the separation was not routine.

Chapter 2

1. These are the words of Jawaharlal Nehru in a letter written from prison in 1944 at the time of the birth of Indira Gandhi's first child, Nehru's grandson, Rajiv.

Chapter 3

1. The concept of archetypes is among the better known theories developed by C. G. Jung traced to his earliest publication in 1902 (Jung 1959). The meaning of archetype is derived from Greek *archē*, "first," and *typos*, "pattern," "stamp," or "mold," and defined as the original models from which things are formed. It is used in psychology as "patterns thought and imagery that emerge from a collective unconscious of humankind" and in literature as "*primordial images* or *archetypal symbols*" found in recurring myths (Peter Angelus, *Dictionary of Philosophy*, p. 17).

Chapter 5

1. An earlier version of this chapter was published in *Phenomenology and Pedagogy. A Human Science Journal* 2(2):178–87.
2. These birthing beds, with warm oak finish, can be transposed into traditional hospital beds by removing the head and foot boards and lowering the foot of the bed to provide better access to assist with the delivery.

Chapter 6

1. Parts of this section were written in collaboration with Dr. Angeline Martel and presented in a paper, "The language of obstetrics from the experience of birthing,"

at the Canadian Research Institute for the Advancement of Women Conference, November 1985. Used here with the permission of Dr. Angeline Martel and CRIAW.

Chapter 7

1. Neumann (1955) talks about this "loss of the original home." Birth is not only a release into life but is also experienced as a rejection from the uterine paradise.

Chapter 8

1. This story was told during a seminar I attended on Family-Centered Perinatal Care held at the University of Alberta in 1983.
2. Refer to note 1 in Chapter 6 for comments about the discussion of "lateness."
3. The word obstetrics comes from the Latin *obstetrīx* meaning "midwife," but apparently this term derives from the verb *obstāre* which means literally to "stand at, before, or against"—usually with the sense "to oppose, hinder."

Chapter 9

1. I am grateful to Penny Simkin for bringing this poem to my attention.
2. This phrase is attributed to the poet Margaret Atwood. I am grateful for R. Heydemann for sharing it with me.

Bibliography

American Psychological Association. *Publication manual of the American Psychological Association* (3rd ed.). Washington, D.C.

Anderson, Gene Cranston, Marks, Elizabeth A. and Wahlberg, Vivian. (1986). Kangaroo care for premature infants. *American Journal of Nursing.* (July): 807–9.

Angeles, Peter. (1981). *Dictionary of philosophy.* New York: Harper & Row.

Annas, George. (1987). Baby M: Babies (and justice) for sale. *Hastings Center Report* 17(3): 13–5.

Aoki, Ted. (1982). *Towards a dialectic between the conceptual world and the lived world: Transcending instrumentalism in curriculum orientation.* Unpublished paper, University of Alberta.

Arditti, Rita, Klein, Renate, and Minden, Shelley (Eds.). (1984). *Test-tube women* Boston: Pandora Press.

Arendt, Hannah. (1958). *The human condition.* Chicago: The University of Chicago.
———. (1961). The crisis in education. *Between past and future* (pp. 173–96). New York: Viking.

Arms, Suzanne. (1975). *Immaculate deception.* S. Hadley, Mass.: Bergin & Garvey.

Ashford, Janet (Ed.). (1984). *Birth stories: The experience remembered.* New York: The Crossing Press.

Atwood, Margaret. (1985). *The handmaid's tale.* Toronto: McClelland & Stewart.

Bachelard, Gaston. (1969). *The poetics of space.* Boston: Beacon.

Balbus, Isaac. (1982). *Marxism and domination.* New Jersey: Princeton University Press.

Baldursson, Stefan. (1985). *The nature of "at-homeness."* Unpublished paper, Faculty of Education, University of Alberta.

Ballard, Edward. (1978). *Man and technology.* Pittsburgh, Pa.: Duquesne University Press.

Barber, Virginia, and Skaggs, Merrill Maguire. (1975). *The mother person.* New York: Bobbs-Merrill.

Bardwick, Judith. (1971). *The psychology of women: A study of bio-cultural conflicts.* New York: Harper & Row.

Barrett, William. (1978). *The illusion of technique.* New York: Doubleday.

————. (1987). *Death of a soul.* New York: Doubleday.

Barrington, Eleanor. (1985). *Midwifery is catching.* Toronto: NC Press.

Barritt, Loren, et al. (1983). *A handbook for phenomenological research in education.* Ann Arbor: University of Michigan.

Bates, Brian, and Turner, Allison. (1985). Imagery and symbolism in the birth practices of traditional cultures. *Birth* 12(1):24–35.

Baumgarten, Kurt. (1981). The advantages and risks of feto-maternal monitoring. *Journal of Perinatal Medicine* 9: 257–74.

Benjamin, Walter. (1969). The storyteller. In *Illuminations* (pp. 83–109). New York: Schocken.

Benner, Patricia. (1985). Quality of life: A phenomenological perspective on explanation, prediction, and understanding in nursing science. *Advances in Nursing Science* 8(1):1–14.

Benoit, Cecilia. (1983). Midwives and healers: The Newfoundland experience. *Health Sharing* (Winter): 22–6.

————. (1984). *From lay knowledge to medical science: The professionalization of midwifery in 20th century Newfoundland.* Unpublished Dissertation Proposal, Department of Sociology, University of Toronto.

Berger, Peter, and Luckmann, Thomas. (1967). *The social construction of reality: A treatise in the sociology of knowledge.* New York: Anchor Books.

Bergsma, Jurrit, and Thomasma, David. (1982). *Health care: Its psychosocial dimensions.* Pittsburgh: Duquesne University Press.

Bernard, Jessie Shirley. (1974). *The future of motherhood.* New York: Dial Press.

Blum, Alan. (1985). *Self-reflection in the arts and sciences.* Toronto: Humanities.

Blumenfeld, Samuel L. (1975). *The retreat from motherhood.* Boston: Beacon.

Böhme, Gernot. (1984). Midwifery as science: An essay on the relation between scientific and everyday knowledge. In N. Stehr and V. Meja (Eds.). *Society and knowledge* (pp. 365–85). New Jersey: Transaction Books.

Bollnow, Otto. (1974). The objectivity of the humanities and the essence of truth. *Philosophy Today* Spring, 3–17.

————. (1987). *Crisis and new beginnings.* Pittsburgh, Pa.: Duquesne University Press.

Bonica, John. (1975). The nature of pain in partuition. *Clinics in Obstetrics and Gynaecology* 3(2): 499–517.

———. (1984). Labor pain. In P. Wall and R. Melzack (Eds.), *Textbook on pain* (pp. 377–92). New York: Churchill Livingstone.

Boston Women's Health Book Collective (1984). *The new our bodies our selves.* New York: Simon & Schuster.

Boulton, Mary G. (1983). *On becoming a mother.* London: Tavistock.

Brackbill, Yvonne, Rice, June, and Young, Diony. (1984). *Birth trap: The legal lowdown on high-tech obstetrics.* Toronto: C. V. Mosby.

Bradley, Robert A. (1974). *Husband-coached childbirth.* New York: Harper & Row.

Breen, Dana. (1975). *The birth of a first child.* London: Tavistock Publication.

Briffault, Robert. (1927). *The mothers: A study of the origins of sentiments and institutions.* 3 vols. London: George Allen & Unwin.

———. (1931). *The mothers. The matriarchal theory of social origins.* New York: Macmillan.

Brown, Norman. (1966). *Love's body.* New York: Random House.

Brownmiller, Susan. (1984). *Femininity.* New York: Fawcett Columbine.

Buck, Pearl. (1931). *The good earth.* New York: Pocket Books.

Burch, Robert. (1984). *Technology and curriculum: toward a philosophical perspective.* Occasional Paper, no. 27. Department of Secondary Education, University of Alberta.

Buytendijk, Frederik Jacobus Johannes. (1961). *Pain.* London: Hutchinson.

———. (1974). *Prolegomena to an anthropological physiology.* Pittsburgh, Pa.: Duquesne University Press.

Cameron, Anne. (1981). *Daughters of copper woman.* Vancouver: Press Gang Publishers.

Castillejo, Irene. (1974). *Knowing women.* New York: Harper & Row.

CBC (Canadian Broadcasting Corporation). (1983). *Being born.* CBC Transcripts, P.O. Box 500, Station "A," Toronto M5W 1E6.

Chamberlain, David. (1983). *Consciousness at birth: A review of empirical evidence.* California: Chamberlain Publications.

Chamberlain, Mary. (1981). *Old wives' tales: Their history, remedies, and spells.* London: Virago.

Chesler, Phyllis. (1979). *With child: A diary of motherhood.* New York: Thomas Y. Crowell.

Chez, Ronald. (1985). Marketing is identifying and meeting the needs of one's patients. *Birth* 12(1): 39–40.

Chicago, Judy. (1985). *The birth project.* New York: Doubleday.

Chinn, Peggy. (1979). Issues in lowering infant mortality: A call for ethical action. *Advances in Nursing Science* 1(3): 63–78.

Chodorow, Nancy. (1978). *The reproduction of mothering: Psychoanalysis and the sociology of gender.* Berkeley: University of California Press.

Clark, Ann, and Affonso, Dyanne. (1976). *Childbearing: A nursing perspective.* Philadelphia: F.A. Davis.

Cohen, Nancy, and Estner, Lois. (1983). *Silent knife: Cesarean prevention and vaginal birth after cesarean.* S. Hadley, Mass.: Bergin & Garvey.

Colen, B. D. (1986). *Hard choices: Mixed blessings of modern medical technology*. New York: G.P. Putnam.

Coles, Robert, and Coles, Jane Hallowell. (1978). *Women of crisis: Lives of struggle and hope*. New York: Dell.

Colman, Arthur D., and Colman, Libby. (1971). *Pregnancy: The psychological experience*. New York: Herder & Herder.

The compact edition of the Oxford English dictionary. (1971). Vol I & II. Oxford: Oxford University Press.

Corea, Gena. (1985). *The mother machine: Reproductive technologies from artificial insemination to artificial wombs*. New York: Harper & Row.

Courter, Gay. (1981). *The midwife*. New York: New American Library.

Cousins, Norman. (1983). *The healing heart: Antidotes to panic and hopelessness*. New York: W. W. Norton.

Daly, Mary. (1978). *Gyn/Ecology: The metaethics of radical feminism*. Boston: Beacon.

————. (1984). *Pure lust: Elemental feminist philosophy*. Boston: Beacon.

Davis, Mary. (1983). *The evolution of prenatal education: A review of the literature*. Unpublished report, Edmonton Local Board of Health, Edmonton, Alberta.

De Certeau, Michel. (1984). *The practice of everyday life*. Berkeley: University of California Press.

Derrida, Jacques. (1973). *Speech and phenomena, and other essays on Husserl's theory of signs*. Evanston: Northwestern University Press.

Dick-Read, Grant. (1972). *Childbirth without fear*. (4th ed.). New York: Harper and Row.

Dinnerstein, Dorothy. (1976). *The mermaid and the minotaur: Sexual arrangements and human malaise*. New York: Harper & Row.

Donoff, Michel Guy, and Paton, Thomas. (1984). *Pre-pregnancy screening in the physician's office and the school*. Unpublished paper presented to Pre-Pregnancy and Pregnancy Health Education and Care Conference, Edmonton, Alberta.

Dowling, Colette. (1981). *The Cinderella complex: Women's hidden fear of independence*. New York: Summit.

Dowrick, Stephanie, and Grundberg, Sibyl. (Eds.). (1980). *Why children?* New York: Harcourt Brace Jovanovich.

Dreifus, Claudia. (Ed.). (1978). *Seizing our bodies: The politics of women's health*. New York: Vintage.

Dunn, P. M. (1979a). Benefits and hazards of fetal and neonatal monitoring. *Perinatal Medicine*: 258–59. VI European Congress, Vienna.

————. (1979b). Problems associated with fetal monitoring during labour, *Perinatal Medicine*, VI European Congress, Vienna, 270–74.

Eagan, Andrea. B. (1985). *The newborn mother: Stages of her growth*. Toronto: Little, Brown.

EBH (1985). *Report of Edmonton Board of Health*. City of Edmonton, Alberta, Canada.

Edie, James. (1984). Report on phenomenology in America. *Research in Phenomenology* XIV: 233–46.

Edwards, Margot, and Waldorf, Mary. (1984). *Reclaiming birth: History and heroines of American childbirth reform*. New York: Crossing Press.

Ehrenreich, Barbara. (1983). *The hearts of men: American dreams and the flight from commitment*. New York: Doubleday.

Ehrenreich, Barbara, and English, Deirdre. (1973). *Witches, midwives, and nurses: A history of women healers*. New York: Feminist Press.

———. (1979). *For her own good: 150 years of experts' advice to women*. New York: Anchor Press/ Doubleday.

ELBH (1984). *Report of the Edmonton Local Board of Health*. City of Edmonton, Alberta, Canada.

Elkins, Valmai. (1983). *The birth report*. Toronto: Lester & Orpen Dennys.

Ellul, Jacques. (1964). *The technological society*. New York: Random House.

Elshtain, Jean. (1982). Feminist discourse and its discontents: Language, power, and meaning. *Signs* 7(3): 603–21.

Engelmann, George Julius. (1884). *Labor among primitive peoples*. St. Louis: J. H. Chambers.

Ermarth, Michael. (1978). *Wilhelm Dilthey: The critique of historical reason*. Chicago: The University of Chicago Press.

Fabe, Marilyn, amd Wikler, Norma. (1979). *Up against the clock: Career women speak on the choice to have children*. New York: Random House.

Fallaci, Oriana. (1976). *Letter to a child never born*. New York: Washington Square Press.

Fauré, Christine. (1981). The twilight of the goddess, or the intellectual crisis of Freud's feminism. *Signs* 7(1): 71–80.

Field, Peggy-Anne. (Ed.). (1984). *Perinatal nursing*. London: Churchill Livingstone.

———. (1985). The birthing process: where should the emphasis be? *The Canadian Nurse* (September): 46–48.

Field, Peggy-Anne, Campbell, Iris, and Buchan J. (1985) *Parent satisfaction with maternity care in traditional and birthing room settings*. Unpublished Report. Faculty of Nursing, University of Alberta.

Firestone, Shulamith. (1970). *The dialectic of sex*. New York: Bantam.

Foucault, Michel. (1975). *The birth of a clinic: An archeology of medical perception*. New York: Vintage.

———. (1978). *The history of sexuality. vol. I. An introduction*. New York: Vintage.

———. (1983). Afterword: The subject and power. In Dreyfus, H., and Pabinow, P. (Eds.). *Michel Foucault: Beyond structuralism and hermeneutics*. Chicago: The University of Chicago Press.

Frankfort, Ellen. (1972). *Vaginal politics*. New York: Bantam.

Franklin, Ursula. (1984). *Reflection on projects and mega-projects*. Presentation at the Women in Toronto Symposium of the School of Graduate Studies, December 4.

———. (1985). *Will women change technology or will technology change women?* The CRIAW Papers, No. 9, Ottawa.

Freire, Paulo. (1973). *Education for critical consciousness*. New York: Seabury.

———. (1978). *Pedagogy in process*. New York: Seabury.

Friedland, Ronnie, and Kort, Carol. (Eds.). (1981). *The mothers' book. Shared experiences*. Boston: Houghton Mifflin.

Fujita, Mikio. (1985). Modes of waiting. *Phenomenology and Pedagogy* 3(2): 107–15.

Gadamer, Hans-Georg. (1975). *Truth and method*. New York: Seabury.

Gaskin, Ina May. (1977). *Spiritual midwifery*. Summertown, Tennessee: Book Publishing Company.

Geertz, Clifford. (1973). *The interpretation of cultures*. New York: Basic.

Gilligan Carol. (1982). *In a different voice*. Cambridge, Mass.: Harvard University Press.

Goer, Henci, and Euzent, Vivian. (1984). Veteran childbirth educators: Are they providing quality services? *Birth* 11(2):109–10.

Goldsmith, Judith. (1984). *Childbirth wisdom: From the world's oldest societies*. New York: Congdon & Weed.

Graham, Harvey. (1960). *Eternal Eve: The mysteries of birth and the customs that surround it*. Toronto: Hutchinson of London.

Grant, George. (1969). *Technology and empire: Perspectives on North America*. Toronto: House of Anansi.

Green, Joy. (1985). Family birthing: what a difference a shift makes! *The Canadian Nurse* 81(9): 40–43.

Greene Maxine. (1978). *Landscapes of learning*. New York: Teachers College Press.

Greer, Germaine. (1984). *Sex and destiny: The politics of human fertility*. Toronto: General Publishing Group.

Griffin, Susan. (1978). *Woman and nature: The roaring inside her*. San Francisco: Harper Colophon.

———. (1981). *Pornography and silence: Culture's revenge against nature*. New York: Harper & Row.

———. (1982). The way of all ideology. *Signs* 7(3): 641–60.

Grumet, Madeleine. (1981). Conception, contradiction, and curriculum. *Journal of Curriculum Theorizing* 3(3): 287–98.

Habermas, Jürgen. (1968). *Knowledge and human interests*. Boston: Beacon.

Haire, Doris. (1972). *The culture warping of childbirth*. Seattle: International Childbirth Education Association.

Harrison, Michelle. (1982). *A woman in residence*. New York: Random House.

Haverkamp, Albert, et al. (1976). The evaluation of continuous fetal heart rate monitoring in high-risk pregnancy. *American Journal of Obstetrics and Gynecology* 125(3): 310–20.

Haverkamp Albert, and Orleans, Miriam. (1983). An assessment of electronic fetal monitoring. In D. Young (Ed.), *Obstetrical intervention and technology in the 1980s* (pp. 115–34). New York: Haworth Press.

Heckler, Richard. (1984). *The anatomy of change*. Boulder: Shambhala.

Heffner, Elaine. (1978). *Mothering: The emotional experience of motherhood after Freud and feminism*. New York: Doubleday.

Heidegger, Martin. (1962). *Being and time*. New York: Harper & Row.

———. (1971). *On the way to language*. New York: Harper & Row.

———. (1977a). *Basic writings*. New York: Harper & Row.

———. (1977b). *The question concerning technology an and other essays*. New York: Harper & Row.

Hodnett, Ellen. (1982). Patient control during labor. *Journal of Obstetrical and Gynecological Nursing* (March/April): 94–99.

Hoff, Gerard Alan, and Schneiderman, Lawrence J. (1985). Having babies at home: Is it safe? Is it ethical? *Hastings Center Report* 15(6): 19–27.

Hollick, Frederick. (1876). *The matron's manual of midwifery, and the diseases of women during pregnancy and in child bed.* New York: Excelsior.

Hubbard, Ruth. (1984). Personal courage is not enough: Some hazards of childbearing in the 1980's. In R. Arditti, R. Duelli, and S. Minden (Eds.), *Test-tube women* (pp. 331–55). Boston: Pandora Press.

Huebner, Dwayne. (1984). The search for religious metaphors in the language of education. *Phenomenology and Pedagogy* 2(2): 112–23.

Husserl, Edmund. (1970). *The crisis of the European sciences and transcendental phenomenology.* Evanston: Northwestern University Press.

———. (1977). *Cartesian Meditations.* The Hague: Martinus Nijhoff.

ICEA. (1987). *Bookmarks.* Minneapolis: International Childbirth Education Association.

———. (1983). Diagnostic ultrasound in obstetrics. *ICEA News* 22(2).

Ihde, Don. (1971). *Hermeneutic phenomenology: The philosophy of Paul Ricoeur.* Evanston: Northwestern University Press.

———. (1979). *Technics and praxis.* Holland: D. Reidel.

———. (1983). *Existential technics.* Albany: State University of New York Press.

Illich, Ivan. (1976). *Limits to medicine.* London: Marion Boyars.

———. (1978). *The right to useful unemployment and its professional enemies.* London: Marion Boyars.

———. (1981). *Shadow work.* Boston: Marion Boyars.

———. (1982). *Gender.* New York: Pantheon.

Israeloff, Roberta. (1982). *Coming to terms.* New York: Penguin.

Jiménez, Sherry. (1980). *Child bearing: A guide for pregnant parents.* New Jersey: Prentice Hall.

———. (1984). The problem of childbirth educator's personal opinions. *Birth* 11(2): 113.

Johnson, Robert. (1976). *She: Understanding feminine psychology.* New York: Harper and Row.

Jordan, Brigitte. (1980). *Birth in four cultures.* Montreal: Eden Press Women's Publications.

Jung, Carl. (1959). *Four archetypes. Mother/rebirth/spirit/trickster.* (Translated by R.F.C. Hull). Princeton: Princeton University Press.

Kaufmann, Walter Arnold. (1968). *Nietzsche: Philosopher, psychologist, antichrist.* New York: Vintage.

Kelpin, Vangie [Bergum]. (1984). Birthing Pain. *Phenomenology and Pedagogy* 2(2): 178–87.

Kelpin, Vangie [Bergum], and Martel, Angeline. (1984). The language of obstetrics from the experience of birthing. *Women: Images, role-models.* (pp. 150–58). Montreal: Canadian Research Institute for the Advancement of Women.

Kittay, Eva Feder. (1983). Womb envy: An explanatory concept. In Joyce Trebilcot (Ed.), *Mothering. Essays in feminist theory* (pp. 94–128). New Jersey: Rowman & Allanhead.

Kitzinger, Sheila. (1962). *The experience of childbirth.* London: Penguin.

————. (1977). *Giving birth, the parents' emotion in childbirth.* New York: Schocken.

————. (1978). *Women as mothers.* Oxford: Martin Robertson.

————. (1979a). *Birth at home.* New York: Oxford University Press.

————. (1979b). *Education and counseling for childbirth.* New York: Schocken.

————. (1983). *Woman's experience of sex.* New York: G. P. Putnam.

Kitzinger, Sheila, and Davis, John A. (Eds.) (1978). *The place of birth.* Oxford: Oxford Medical Publications.

Kitzinger, Sheila, and Simkin, Penny. (Eds.) (1984). *Episiotomy and the second stage of labor.* Seattle: Pennypress.

Klaus, Marshall, and Kennell, John. (1976). *Maternal-infant bonding.* St. Louis: C. V. Mosby.

Kloosterman, G. (1979). Intrapartum benefits and hazards of monitoring. *Perinatal Medicine*: 279–83. VI European Congress, Vienna.

Kohák, Erazim. (1978). *Idea and experience: Edmund Husserl's project of phenomenology in ideas I.* Chicago: The University of Chicago Press.

Kotre, John. (1984). *Outliving the self: Generativity and the interpretation of lives.* Baltimore: Johns Hopkins University Press.

Kramarae, Cheris, and Treichler, Paula. (1985). *A feminist dictionary.* Boston: Pandora.

Kristeva, Julia. (1981). Women's time. *Signs* 7(1): 13–35.

Kvale, Steinar. (1984). The qualitative research interview: A phenomenological and hermeneutical mode of understanding. *Journal of Phenomenological Psychology* 14(2): 171–96.

Laing, R. D. (1982). *The voice of experience.* London: Penguin.

Lang, Raven. (Speaker). (1985). *Midwifery tradition: Roots and renewal.* (Cassette Recording). Midwifery Conference, San Francisco.

Langan, Thomas. (1984). Phenomenology and appropriation. *Phenomenology and Pedagogy* 2(2): 101–11.

Langer, Susanne. (1973). *Philosophy in a new key.* Cambridge: Harvard University Press.

Lazarre, Jane. (1976). *The mother knot.* New York: Dell.

Leboyer, Frederick. (1975). *Birth without violence.* New York: Knopf.

Leder, Drew. (1984). Medicine and paradigms of embodiment. *The Journal of Medicine and Philosophy* 9(1): 29–44.

Leifer, Myra. (1980). *Psychological effects of pregnancy: A study of first pregnancy.* New York: Praeger.

Levinas, Emmanuel. (1981). *Otherwise than being or beyond essence* (A. Lingris, Trans.). Boston: Martinus Nijhof.

Levine, Carol, Bermel, Joyce, and Homer, Paul. (1987). Biomedical ethics: A multinational view. *Hastings Center Report* 17 (3, Special Supplement): 1–36.

Lincoln, Bruce. (1981). *Emerging from the chrysalis. Studies in rituals of women's initiation.* Cambridge, Mass.: Harvard University Press.

Lozoff, Betsy, et al. (1977). The mother-newborn relationship: Limits of adaptability. *The Journal of Pediatrics* 91: 1–12.

Luckmann, Thomas. (Ed). (1978). *Phenomenology and sociology: Selected readings.* Middlesex: Penguin Books.

————. (1983). Common sense, science and specialization of knowledge. *Phenomenology and Pedagogy* 1(1): 59–73.

McCarthy, T. A. (1973). A theory of communication competence. *Philosophy of the Social Sciences* 3: 135–56.

McDermott, John. (1986). The stethoscope as talisman: Medical technology and loneliness. *AARN Newsletter* 42(2): 21–24.

Macfarlene Aidan. (1977). *The psychology of childbirth*. Cambridge: Harvard University Press.

McKay, Susan. (1982). *Humanizing maternity services through family-centered care*. Minneapolis, Minn.: International Childbirth Education Association.

MacPherson, Katherine. (1981). Menopause as disease: The social construction of a metaphor. *Advances in Nursing Science* 3(2): 95–113.

————. (1983). Feminist methods: a new paradigm from nursing research. *Advances in Nursing Science* 5(2): 17–25.

McRoberts, Viviene. (1984). Miracle on 87 St. *The Edmonton Journal*, Jan. 15. Alberta, Canada.

Mahler, Halfden. (1981). The meaning of "health for all by the year 2000." *World Health Forum* 2(1): 5–22.

Mannheim, Karl. (1936). *Ideology and utopia*. New York: Harcourt, Brace & World.

Marcel, Gabriel. (1978). *Homo viator: Introduction to a metaphysic of hope*. Gloucester, Mass: Peter Smith.

Martel, Angeline, and Peterat, Linda. (in press). A hope for hopelessness: *Womanness at the margin in schools*. *Journal of Curriculum Theorizing*.

Meerloo, Joost. (1960). *The dance*. New York: Chilton.

Mehl, Lewis E., Peterson, Gail H., Whitt, Michael, and Hawes, Warren E. (1977). Outcomes of elective home births: A series of 1,146 cases. *The Journal of Reproductive Medicine* 19: 281–90.

Meinhart, Noreen, and McCaffery, Margo. (1983). *Pain: A nursing approach to assessment and analysis*. Norwalk, Conn.: Appleton-Century-Crofts.

Meltzer, David. (Ed). (1981). *Birth, an anthology of ancient texts, songs, prayers, and stories*. San Francisco: North Point.

Melzack, Ronald. (1973). *The puzzle of pain*. Middlesex: Penguin.

Melzack, Ronald, Taenzer, Paul, Feldman, Parle, and Kinch, Robert. (1980). Labour is still painful after prepared childbirth training. *Canadian Medical Association Journal* 4(125): 357–63.

Menendez-Bauer, C., Arroyo, L., Reina, L., Menendez, S., and Zammariego, J. (1979). Monitoring and maternal posture. *Perinatal Medicine*: 294–95. VI European Congress, Vienna.

Merleau-Ponty, Maurice. (1962). *Phenomenology of perception*. London: Routledge & Kegan Paul.

————. (1964). *The primacy of perception*. Evanston: Northwestern University Press.

————. (1968). *The visible and the invisible*. Evanston: Northwestern University Press.

Miller, Jean Baker. (1976). *Toward a new psychology of women*. Boston: Beacon.

Mills, Karen, Paddon, Doreen, Edwards, Joyce, and Kelpin, Vangie [Bergum]. (1982). *Survey of knowledge and interests of registrants in early prenatal classes*. Unpublished Report, Edmonton Local Board of Health.

Misgeld, Deiter. (1983). Phenomenology, social science, and the social service professions. The case for the integration of phenomenology, hermeneutics, and critical theory. (A reply to Luckmann and Giorgi). *Phenomenology and Pedagogy* 1(2): 195–214.

Molfese, Victoria., Sunshine, Philip, and Bennett, Allen. (1982). Reactions of Women to intrapartum fetal monitoring. *Obstetrics and Gynecology* 59(6): 705–09.

Montagu, Ashley. (1971). *Touching: The human significance of the skin.* New York: Columbia University Press.

Morgan, George A. (1941). *What Nietzsche means.* New York: Harper & Row.

Morgan, Robin. (1977). *Going too far.* New York: Random House.

———. (1984). *The anatomy of freedom: Feminism, physics and global politics.* New York: Anchor Books/Doubleday.

Morris, William. (Ed.). (1978). *The American heritage dictionary of the English language.* Boston: Houghton Mifflin.

Murray, Jessica. (1983). Elsa's birth. In P. O'Mara McMahon, M. Cohen, K. Kaiser-Cook, and K. Fischer (Eds.), *Mother Poet* (p. 34). Albuquerque, N.M.: Mothering Publication.

NDP. (1983). *Domiciliary midwives and homebirths.* Alberta: NDP.

Nelson, Margaret. (1983). Working-class women, middle-class women, and models of childbirth. *Social Problems* 30(3): 284–97.

Neumann, Erich. (1955). *The great mother: An analysis of the archetype.* Princeton: Princeton University Press.

Newton, Niles. (1955). *Maternal emotions.* Pennsylvania: Paul B. Hoeber.

Nightingale, Florence. (1859/1980). *Notes on nursing: What it is, and what it is not.* New York: Churchill Livingstone.

Novak, Michael. (1978). Autobiography and Story. *Ascent of the mountain, flight of the dove* (pp. 43–87). San Francisco: Harper & Row.

Oakley, Ann. (1979). A case of maternity: Paradigms of women as maternity cases. *Signs* 4(4): 607–31.

———. (1980a). *Becoming a mother.* New York: Schocken.

———. (1980b). *Women confined: Towards a sociology of childbirth.* London: Schocken.

———. (1984). *The captured womb: A history of the medical care of pregnant women.* Great Britain: Oxford Publishing Services.

———. (1986a). The history of ultrasonography in obstetrics. *Birth* 13(1): 8–13.

———. (1986b). *Telling the truth about Jerusalem.* New York: Basil Blackwell.

O'Brien, Mary. (1981). *The politics of reproduction.* Boston: Routledge & Kegan Paul.

Odent, Michel. (1981). The evolution of obstetrics at Pithiviers. *Birth and the Family Journal* 1(8): 7–15.

———. (1984a). *Birth reborn.* New York: Pantheon.

———. (1984b). *Entering the world: The de-medicalization of childbirth.* New York: Marion Boyars.

Olson, Carol. (1986). *How can we understand the life of illness?* Unpublished doctoral dissertation, University of Alberta.

Omery, Anna. (1983). Phenomenology. A method for nursing research. *Advances in Nursing Science* 5(2): 49–63.

Panuthos, Claudia. (1984). *Transformation through birth.* S. Hadley, Mass.: Bergin & Garvey.

Parse, Rosemarie, Coyne, A. Barbara, and Smith, Mary Jane. (1985). *Nursing research: Qualitative methods.* Bowie, Md.: Brady Communications.

Pearce, Joseph Chilton. (1977). *Magical child.* Toronto: Bantam.

Pelletier, Kenneth. (1979). *Holistic medicine: From stress to optimal health.* New York: Delacort Press/Seymour Lawrence.

Peterson, Gayle. (1981). *Birthing normally: A personal growth approach to childbirth.* Berkeley: Mindbody Press.

Peterson, Karen J. (1983). Technology as a last resort in home birth: The work of lay midwives. *Social Problems* 30(3): 272–83.

Phillips, Celeste R., and Anzalone, Joseph T. (1982). *Fathering participation in labor and birth.* Toronto: C. V. Mosby.

Polakow, Valerie. (1984). Reflections on pedagogy, research and praxis. *Phenomenology and Pedagogy* 2(1): 29–35.

Polanyi, Michael. (1958). *Personal knowledge.* Chicago: University of Chicago Press.

———. (1969). *Knowing and being.* Chicago: University of Chicago Press.

Pritchard, Jack A., MacDonald, Paul, and Gant, Norman. (1985). *Williams Obstetrics.* Norwalk, Conn.: Appleton-Century-Crofts.

Rapoport, Rhona, Rapoport, Robert, and Strelitz, Ziona. (1977). *Fathers, mothers, and others.* London: Routledge & Kegan Paul.

Rapp, Rayna. (1984). XYLO: A true story. In R. Arditti, R. Duelli, and S. Minden (Eds.), *Test-tube women* (pp. 313–28). Boston: Pandora.

Reese, Lyn, Wilkinson, Jean, and Koffpelman, Phyllis. (Eds.). (1983). *I'm on my way running. Women speak of coming of age.* New York: Avon.

Rich, Adrienne. (1976). *Of women born.* New York: Bantam.

———. (1978). The theft of childbirth. In C. Dreifus (Ed.), *Seizing our bodies: The politics of women's health* (pp. 146–63). New York: Vintage.

Ricoeur, Paul. (1973a). The task of hermeneutics. *Philosophy Today* 17(2): 112–28.

———. (1973b). The hermeneutic function of distanciation. *Philosophy Today* 17(2): 129–41.

Roberts, Helen. (Ed.). *Women, health, and reproduction.* London: Routledge & Kegan Paul.

Romney, Mona, and White, V.G.L. (1984). Current practices in labour. In P.-A. Field (Ed.). *Perinatal nursing* (pp. 63–80). London: Churchill Livingstone.

Rorty, Richard. (1979). *Philosophy and the mirror of nature.* Princeton, Princeton University Press.

Rothman, Barbara. (1982). *Giving birth: Alternatives in childbirth.* New York: Penguin.

———. (1983). Midwives in transition: The structure of a clinical revolution. *Social Problems* 30(3): 262–71.

———. (1984). The meaning of choice in reproductive technology. In R. Arditti, R. Duelli, and S. Minden (Eds.), *Test-tube women* (pp. 23–33), Boston: Pandora.

———. (1985). Beyond risks and rates in obstetrical care. *Birth* 12(2): 91–94.

———. (1987). *Tentative pregnancy.* New York: Penguin.

Rubin, Reva. (1984). *Maternal identity and the maternal experience.* New York: Springer.

Ruddick, Sara. (1983). Maternal Thinking. In J. Trebilcot (Ed.), *Mothering. Essays in feminist theory* (pp. 211–30). New Jersey: Rowman & Allanhead.

Ruether, Rosemary. (1983). *To change the world. Christology and cultural criticism.* New York: Crossroad.

Russell, Anne, and Fitzgibbons, Patricia. (1982). *Career and conflict. A woman's guide to making life choices.* New Jersey: Prentice Hall.

Sartre, Jean-Paul. (1956). *Being and nothingness.* New York: Washington Square Press.

Scarry, Elaine. (1985). *The body in pain: The making and unmaking of the world.* New York: Oxford University Press.

Seiden, Anne. (1978). The sense of mastery in the childbirth experience. In M. Notman, and C. Nadelson (Eds.). *The woman patient: Medical and psychological interfaces.* (pp. 87–105). New York: Plenum Press.

Sesonske, Alexander, and Fleming, Noel. (1965). *Plato's Meno.* California: Wadsworth.

Shapiro, H. Svi. (1983). Educational research, social change and the challenge to methodology: A Study in the sociology of knowledge. *Phenomenology and Pedagogy* 1(2): 127–39.

Shaver, Joan. (1986). High touch nursing in a high tech world. *Canadian Nurse* 82(5): 16–19.

Shearer, Beth. (1984). Whose birth, whose body, whose baby is it? *Birth* 11(3): 174–75.

Shearer, Madeleine. (1984). Reconsidering the "market model" in obstetrics. Part 1. *Birth* 11(4): 213–14.

Shearer, Madeleine, and Estes, Milton. (1985). A critical review of the recent literature on postterm pregnancy and a look at women's experiences. *Birth* 12(2): 95–111.

Sherard, Jain Nyborg. (1980). *Mother warrior pilgrim: A personal chronicle.* New York: Andrews & McMeel.

Shields, Donna. (1978). Maternal reactions to fetal monitoring. *American Journal of Nursing* 3: 2110–12.

Shorter, Edward. (1982). *A history of women's bodies.* New York: Basic.

Silverman, Hugh. (1984). Phenomenology: From hermeneutics to deconstruction. *Research in Phenomenology* 14: 19–34.

Simkin, Penny. (1983). Amniotomy. In D. Young (Ed.). *Obstetrical intervention and technology in the 1980s* (pp. 103–14). New York: Haworth.

Simkin, Penny, Whalley, Janet, and Keppler, Ann. (1984). *Pregnancy, childbirth and the newborn: A complete guide for expectant parents.* Minnesota: Meadowbrook.

Simonton, Carl, Simonton, Stephanie, and Creighton, James. (1978). *Getting well again.* Los Angeles: J. P. Tarcher.

Smith, David. (1983). *The meaning of children in the lives of adults: A hermeneutic study.* Unpublished doctoral dissertation. University of Alberta.

———. (1984). Living with children. *Phenomenology and Pedagogy* 2(3): 287–92.

Smith, Dorothy. (1980). An analysis of ideological structures and how women are excluded: Considerations for academic women. In J. Grayson (Ed.). *Class, state, ideology, and change.* Toronto: Holt, Rinehart & Winston.

Sorel, Nancy. (1984). *Ever since Eve: Personal reflections on childbirth.* New York: Oxford University Press.

Stainton, Colleen. (1985). *Origins of attachment: Culture and cue sensitivity.* Unpublished doctoral dissertation. University of California, San Francisco.

Stanley, Liz, and Wise, Sue. (1983). *Breaking out: Feminist consciousness and feminist research.* London: Routledge & Kegan Paul.

Starkman, Monica. (1977). Fetal monitoring: Psychologic consequences and management recommendations. *Obstetrics and Gynecology* 50(4): 500–04.

Starr, Paul. (1982). *The social transformation of American medicine.* New York: Basic.

Starrett, B. (1982). The metaphors of power. In Spretnak, C. (Ed.). *The politics of women's spirituality* (pp. 185–93). New York: Anchor.

Stewart, David, and Stewart Lee. (Eds.). (1976). *Safe alternatives in childbirth.* North Carolina: The National Association of Parents and Professionals for Safe Alternatives in Childbirth.

Stewart, Nancy. (1986). Women's view of ultrasonography in obstetrics. *Birth* 13(1): 39–43.

Storch, Janet. (1982). *Ethical and legal issues of human reproduction.* A background paper prepared for the fifth program in ACCESS television series Medical/Legal Issues. Edmonton.

Suransky, Valerie. (1982). *The erosion of childhood.* Chicago: The University of Chicago Press.

Sweet, Lois. (1983). Series on childbirth. *Edmonton Journal,* Feb.-Apr. Edmonton, Alberta.

Thacker, Stephen. (1986). Research strategies for the use of imaging ultrasound as an obstetrical screening tool. *Birth* 13(1):44–47.

Thacker, Stephen, and Banta, H. David. (1983). Benefits and risks of episiotomy. In D. Young (Ed.) *Obstetrical intervention and technology in the 1980s.* New York: Haworth Press.

Trebilcot, Joyce. (Ed.). (1983). *Mothering. Essays in feminist theory.* New Jersey: Rowman & Allanheld.

Tucker, Susan. (1979). *Fetal monitoring and its fetal assessment in high-risk pregnancy.* St. Louis: C. V. Mosby.

U.S. Department of Human Services. (1984). *Diagnostic ultrasound: Imaging in pregnancy.* NIH Publication No. 84–667.

Valentine, Deborah. (1982). The experience of pregnancy: A developmental process. *Family Relations* 31: 243–48.

Van den Berg, Jon Hendrick. (1972). *The psychology of the sickbed.* Pittsburgh: Duquesne University Press.

———. (1974). *A different existence.* Pittsburgh: Duquesne University Press.

Van Gennep, Arnold. (1960). *The rites of passage.* London: Routledge & Kegan Paul.

Van Manen, Max. (1982). Edifying theory serving the good. *Theory into Practice* 21(3): 44–50.

———. (1984a). *"Doing" phenomenological research and writing: An introduction.* Monograph No. 7, University of Alberta.

———. (1984b). *Action research as a theory of the unique: From pedagogic thoughtfulness to pedagogic tactfulness.* Unpublished manuscript, University of Alberta.

———. (1986a). *The tone of teaching.* Ontario: Scholastic-TAB.

————. (1986b). We need to show how our human science practice is a relation to pedagogy. *Phenomenology and Pedagogy* 4(3)3: 78–93.

Verny, Thomas, and Kelly, John. (1981). *The secret life of the unborn child*. New York: Delta.

Weizenbaum, Joseph. (1976). *Computer power and human reason*. San Francisco: W. H. Freeman.

Wertz, Richard, and Wertz, Dorothy. (1979). *Lying in: A history of childbirth in America*. New York: Schocken.

Wilson, Janet. (1982). *Perspectives on motherhood: A phenomenological study of women's transitions to motherhood*. Unpublished master's thesis, University of Alberta.

Wolkind, Stejem. and Zajicek, Eva. (Eds.). (1981). *Pregnancy: A psychological and social study*. Toronto: Academic Press.

Woodman, Marion. (1980). *Addiction to perfection*. Toronto: Inner City Books.

————. (1985). *The pregnant virgin: A process of psychological transformation*. Toronto: Inner City Books.

Young, Diony. (1978).*Bonding*. Minneapolis, Minn.: ICEA.

————. (Ed.). (1983). *Obstetrical intervention and technology in the 1980's*. New York: Haworth.

————. (1987). Crisis in obstetrics—the management of labor. *International Journal of Childbirth Education* 2(3): 13–15.

Young, Iris. (1984). Pregnant embodiment: Subjectivity and alienation. *The Journal of Medicine and Philosophy* 9(1): 45–60.

Zaner, Richard. (1970). *The way of phenomenology*. New York: Pegasus.

————. (1971). *The problem of embodiment: Some contributions to a phenomenology of the body*. The Hague: Martinus Nijhoff.

INDEX